'For the first time, we have a systematic enquiry into essences, how they are made, used and how they affect us. But the book is so much more: a full application of the science of subtle medicine with clarification and advice for good practice.'

– *Julian Barnard, Healing Herbs*

'Sue guides us from the basic elements of an essence, the water of life, with its unique properties and ability to flow, to the myriad of different types of essences now made across the globe.'

– *from the Foreword by Tony Pinkus, Director,*
Ainsworths Homeopathic Pharmacy, London

of related interest

The Practitioner's Encyclopedia of Flower Remedies
The Definitive Guide to All Flower Essences, their Making and Uses
Clare G. Harvey
ISBN 978 1 84819 173 0
eISBN 978 0 85701 126 8

Principles of Bach Flower Remedies
What it is, how it works, and what it can do for you
Stefan Ball
ISBN 978 1 84819 142 6
eISBN 978 0 85701 120 6

The Compassionate Practitioner
How to create a successful and rewarding practice
Jane Wood
ISBN 978 1 84819 222 5
eISBN 978 0 85701 170 1

Colour Healing Manual
The Complete Colour Therapy Programme
Pauline Wills
ISBN 978 1 84819 165 5
eISBN 978 0 85701 131 2

Fragrance and Wellbeing
Plant Aromatics and Their Influence on the Psyche
Jennifer Peace Rhind
ISBN 978 1 84819 090 0
eISBN 978 0 85701 073 5

THE ESSENCE PRACTITIONER

CHOOSING AND USING FLOWER AND OTHER ESSENCES

SUE LILLY

Foreword by Tony Pinkus
Introduction by Simon Lilly

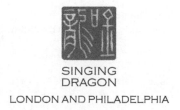

SINGING
DRAGON

LONDON AND PHILADELPHIA

Flower illustrations by Simon Lilly on pages 10, 18, 74 and
185 reproduced with kind permission of the artist.

This edition published in 2015
by Singing Dragon
an imprint of Jessica Kingsley Publishers
73 Collier Street
London N1 9BE, UK
and
400 Market Street, Suite 400
Philadelphia, PA 19106, USA

First edition published by Tree Seer Publications in 2014

www.singingdragon.com

Library of Congress Cataloging in Publication Data
Lilly, Sue.
 The essence practitioner : choosing and using flower and
other essences / Sue Lilly ; Foreword by Tony
Pinkus.
   pages cm
 Includes bibliographical references.
 ISBN 978-1-84819-250-8 (alk. paper)
 1. Aromatherapy. 2. Essences and essential oils--Therapeutic
use. I. Pinkus, Tony, writer of preface. II.
Title.
 RM666.A68L54 2015
 615.3'219--dc23
                    2014021431

British Library Cataloguing in Publication Data
A CIP catalogue record for this book is available from the British Library

ISBN 978 1 84819 250 8
eISBN 978 0 85701 198 5

Printed and bound in Great Britain

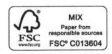

CONTENTS

FOREWORD

'There are more things in heaven and earth, Horatio, than are dreamt of in your philosophy' *Hamlet* (1.5.167–8), Shakespeare. Spirit invests life and character in every being and thing, the essence of the being is its spirit and the qualities of that spirit are captured in the essence it imbues. Essences represent that invisible quality of spirit that represent the life of a being and gathering essences for healing purposes is an ancient practice.

Modern medicine eschews (is apt to dismiss) essences as placebos, because its blinkered view of science is limited to physical representation alone. However, if man is the hardware consider, dear reader, who created the software and where does this reside? Where does the instruction come for each cell to activate its DNA to create the proteins that build material life? Who makes your decisions, who is doing the thinking and feeling in your being?

Sue Lilly has produced within these pages, a very comprehensive and grounded encyclopaedic approach to essences and their manufacture. Many books on this subject lose a wider audience by their esoteric style, but Sue's book benefits greatly from her scientific background, astrological training and broad knowledge and experience of essences. Her many years as a teacher of essence use make this book a sound reference text and a pleasure to read. I have had the great pleasure to work with Sue as the Chairman of BAFEP (British Association of Flower Essence Producers) for many years and I am aware that everything she undertakes is done thoroughly well. This book is no exception and I commend it wholeheartedly as I know it will be a boon to practitioners from all walks of life.

Nothing can, or indeed, should replace personal experience; however, in the search for this you are safely guided by the wealth of knowledge Sue has accumulated in her many years of practice. This book is written from her personal experience spanning many decades. She brings the esoteric into practical use with simple cogent explanation. She takes a pragmatic approach to the whole subject of essences from fundamental principles, to manufacture and administration.

Sue guides us from the basic elements of an essence, the water of life, with its unique properties and ability to flow, to the myriad of different types of essences now made across the globe. She describes the methods in her down-to-earth way and follows this with the practical use in an equally simple practical manner.

Who is this booked aimed at? Primarily practitioners who wish to improve their knowledge of practising with and prescribing essences. I would suggest it is essential reading, as a core curriculum reference text, for anyone studying essences and their use. Sue describes the many ways of using essences, together with the principles and practice of a diverse range of practice styles. Her book is inclusive of all essences rather than being limited to a particular genre of essence, and her chapter on techniques for testing the patient by a plethora of simply learned physical dowsing techniques is extremely valuable to any practitioner.

This book is, in summary, a very pragmatic and essential addition to the library of any practitioner expanding their knowledge on essences in general.

Tony Pinkus
May 2014

ACKNOWLEDGEMENTS

Thanks to Brian Parsons, Tony Pinkus and Simon H. Lilly for their support in finally getting this book into print, and to Simon for the plant images!

Thanks to Steve Mason for his example on the discernment of Lithium Quartz gem essence.

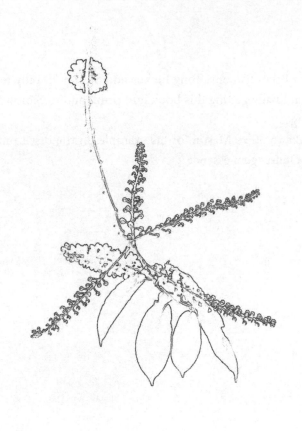

PREFACE

This book provides information for people new to essence use; it introduces new ideas for those who have experience, and it provides an opportunity to broaden the whole concept of what essences are, how they are made and how they can be used.

This book also offers the opportunity to reassess and re-evaluate the role and application of essences. Sometimes it is easy and comfortable to stay with what is considered traditional as this is safe, familiar and conveys some certainty. Here, beliefs that have anchored essences and their use in the past have not been left behind, but have been augmented by insights and new discoveries.

This is not a 'cookbook' for 'this essence does this'. This is a book for possible ways to use any essences from any producer, including ones made personally. It also gives strategies for discerning what an essence does for an individual, regardless of what the producer or an author has written about it.

It is very apparent when reading about essences that have been with us for nearly 100 years that defining something, limits something.

Pine/Scot's Pine (*Pinus sylvestris*) is a prime example. The keyword that has become associated with Pine essence is 'guilt'. If a client feels guilty then this is the essence to use. However by using the techniques in this book it is possible to broaden out the understanding of any essence.

Taking a personal look at pine essence:

Colour key of the flowers: red/pink.

Colour key of the essence: indigo (dowsed/muscle/tested).

Chakra key: brow (dowsed/muscle/tested).

Area of the body: relaxation in the heart chakra (dowsed/muscle/tested and information from knowledge of the essential oil).

Pooling the correspondences from these, the idea of easing guilt becomes clearer.

By working on the heart chakra, emotional tension is released and boundaries become more secure. However the colour key and chakra key hint at increased insight (brow chakra) and the ability to stand back from a situation (indigo), both bringing greater understanding and a broader view. The colour of the flowers hints at the ability to take action (red) and the support to be kinder to and less harsh on oneself (pink).

How to use essences is also changing. In 1997 at the International Flower Essence Conference at Findhorn, Simon and I presented an immersion in essence energy through slides, symbols, colour, sound and essences sprayed in the auditorium for the trees Yew and Elm. This was the first time we had gone 'public' with our work and our ideas of how essences could be presented and used. It was a hit! Judy Hall referred to it as 'tripping with trees!'

At the first flower essence gathering in 1998 at Leiston Abbey, it was also recognised that the future of essences lay in the hands of the many people present and in their ability to pass on their knowledge and skills to the coming generations. It was acknowledged that there were many people making essences in the UK, and that as a community we could work towards securing a future for both ourselves and essences.

This book is part of that vision. I started it in 1998 and picked it up at various points from then until 2008 when it lay dormant until 2013. It has always had a life of its own, so maybe its time has come!

INTRODUCTION

Flower essences began at a time when they seemed just another expression of the traditional uses of herbs and the benefits of homoeopathy were not so doubted as they are today.

Dr Bach came from an era where at least some notable and erudite academics felt able to support research on the fringes of scientific knowledge through such bodies as the Theosophical Society and the Society for Psychical Research. Religion, as well as science, was still a foundation stone of Western culture, tempered by the practical discoveries of the rapidly developing chemical and physical sciences.

Today, essences are often associated with seemingly disparate, but thematically linked therapeutic models variously called 'energy medicine', 'vibrational medicine' and 'resonance therapy'. Those who are familiar with these modalities and their terminologies often fail to appreciate how uncomfortably these terms sit in the minds of many people.

Words live and breathe in their own specific and rarified environments. Take a word from its familiar, accepted and understood context and it soon breaks down, losing the clarity of its defined edges, even transforming into contradictory meanings.

'Energy' seems such a clear-cut, ordinary word, yet it turns out to be profoundly uncertain and diaphanous. In its everyday, familiar context 'energy' is not a thing at all, but an observed effect. One gets energy from food, one loses energy and becomes tired. We can have the energy to do countless things, yet lose it unaccountably. Energy, in these contexts, is an everyday, subjective experience. Energy equates to the motivation or fuel to get things done.

In the terminology of science, 'energy' still means this input of activating force, but it becomes associated specifically with the electromagnetic (EM) spectrum. The nature of this energy, its substance, eludes us, but we could name it 'light'. The electromagnetic spectrum extends from very short wavelengths (labelled gamma radiation), to very long wavelengths (labelled radio waves), with visible light about in the middle of the range. Whether a wave is a nanometre long or millions of miles long, all electromagnetic radiation travels at the speed of light.

However, the source of all electromagnetic radiations is always matter. All matter continuously absorbs and radiates EM frequencies, the signature determined by the internal structure of the matter concerned.

So matter is the source of 'energy', but when we probe deeper into the nature of matter, (molecules, atoms, atomic particles, subatomic particles) all we find is energy, which instead of expanding outwards in linear waveforms, is fixed in orbital relationships that constantly change depending on how much other energy is emitted or absorbed.

One definition of light is mass-energy that only exists when it is moving very fast, whilst matter is mass-energy that can exist staying still. It is so difficult to define what 'energy' is, because there is nothing that is not energy, pure and simple. All we seem to be able to do is define the qualities of different aspects of this pervading something that is nothing.

Contemporary scientific language has done a sterling job of avoiding spiritual and metaphysical metaphors in its finer and finer explorations of matter and its energy states, but these surely lurk just below the surface of its measured, rational explanation for how everything appears to work. It has been the independent philosophers and explorers of awareness, as well as energy healers, who have taken on board a more overtly metaphysical model of reality. One of the models has been the Six Systems of Hindu Philosophy, specifically the branches of Vaisheshika and Sankhya, which analyse and categorise the processes of creation and manifestation from the most subtle states to the most material. The practical expressions of these theories relating to the human body are found within the branch of Yoga, and it is from here that the Theosophists first popularised the system of chakras and subtle bodies.

We should remember that Dr Bach called his own system of flower remedies 'soul medicine', and that he designed the system of essences to interact with what he perceived as underlying emotional patterns that set up predilections for disease states.

One of the fundamental characteristics of energy medicine is its focus on the individual as a dynamic equilibrium of forces. Matter is what our biology experiences as holding patterns, temporarily localised in time and space. Energy medicine includes those techniques that seem to work upon these energy fields. They all, to one degree or another, fall outside parameters that mainstream science feels comfortable looking at, but to some significant statistical degree they benefit, or seem to benefit, those who choose to use them.

Whilst orthodox physics accepts that electromagnetic forces constitute all levels of existence, orthodox medical philosophy prefers to stick to a more mechanistic 'things are real and solid' model. They, understandably, feel more comfortable with a terminology of cause and effect, measurability and repeatability. A flower essence whose active elements cannot even be identified by the most finely calibrated analytical device will always remain at the limits of believability.

The analogy of music, and particularly the modern technologies that allow us to hear recorded music, can help us to understand how essences might work. First, these carriers, namely, MP3 players, CDs, radios, give no external clues to the information they contain. They require an appropriate translating device or energy input to reproduce the recorded material. An essence is also a recording of vibration, held within a neutral material, usually water. The human body and its sensitivity to very small fluctuations of energy is the player that activates and responds to the recording.

Music can be categorised by the general emotional response it evokes. Certain notes, intervals, scales and instruments are recognised as sad, melancholy, joyful, stirring and so on. Yet at a personal level, the summoning of these emotions might at one time be welcomed and appropriate and at other times unsuitable and irritating. The same can be said about essences. It is possible to broadly define the qualities of an essence, but not how the individual will interact with an essence at any one time. This is why a client-based approach using subtle assessment skills and intuition can often prove to be the most effective way to select appropriate essences.

Sound and music is a rather easily measured vibration of waves that interacts with our primary sense mechanisms. Vibrational medicine says that there are many other things that can interact beneficially with the human system and has developed ways of externalising the sensing mechanisms of the body to demonstrate, at least to itself, that these effects can be detected using dowsing, muscle testing and intuitive choice.

Vibrational medicine is largely 'irrational' in that it must rely on such processes that are alien to the conscious mind and its habitual ways of working. Only a minute proportion of information from the external energetic world gets to attract the attention of the conscious mind. Much less than 1 per cent of internal and external phenomena passes through the various filters of the nervous system and brain to impinge upon our waking consciousness. Yet this consciousness, this awareness that we call 'me', this language-using, storytelling part of the human system is not really in control of the body, or the mind, as a whole. Though it might like to think of itself as in the driving seat, it is more akin to a passenger with limited choices of perception and action. Effective essence practitioners are those who have trained themselves to pay attention both to the client and to their own deep minds.

All things are affected by the electromagnetic spectrum. Those things (that we call 'matter') are, it turns out, also just made of interactions of other electromagnetic forces. Weak and strong forces 'hold together' or interact to form atoms. But, when examined, the solidity of atoms dissolves into smaller and smaller packets of an electromagnetic nature, which we call energy. So this interaction of forces seems to be nothing but actions and functions acting on other actions and functions. If this is indeed reality, then it might not seem so far-fetched that the judicious application of an essence might bring about a quantum (energy) shift in the life experience and well-being of a human being.

Simon H. Lilly
May 2014

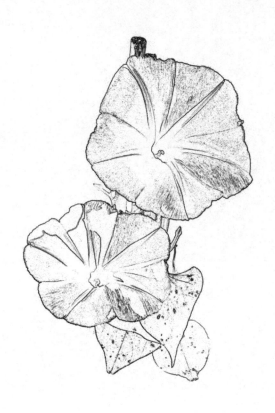

PART ONE

CHOOSING AND USING ESSENCES

CHAPTER 1

WHAT ARE ESSENCES?

In the autumn of 1997 we were invited to the International Flower Essence Conference at Findhorn in Scotland where we were able to present some of the aspects of this work with tree essences and tree spirits. It was a good experience to meet other people making and using essences. After our return, however, we realised that no-one seems to have addressed some of the most fundamental questions regarding essences, perhaps because they do not have answers at the moment. The most basic of questions: putting aside the definitions, the stock phrases, the jargon, what is it that we believe enters into the water? What is the nature of the essence? What is the 'energy'? What is the 'vibration'? What turns it into 'energy medicine'?

Excerpt from *Tree: Essence of Healing*, Simon and Sue Lilly, 1999.

No longer are essences simply being made from flowers as they used to be. Now essences are being made of special environments, of seasonal events like solstices, of sea animals, of shells. The thought arises: if I lie in a pool of spring water in sunlight for a couple of hours is that water now imbued with 'essence of me'? Does it have my energetic imprint? Is it a vibrational healing tool?

Is there any difference between 'essence', 'spirit', 'soul', 'vibratory energy pattern' or 'signature'? Or are we using different words to explain the same phenomenon? Is a 'spirit' a localised semi-permanent folding of the universal field? Is it an energy signature? Is the 'spirit' in the essence? Or is the essence like a footprint, fingerprint or key to the spirit?

Some essence makers shared their experiences at Findhorn of making an essence, describing seeing lines of light, force or energy being carried from the plant to the water via the cut flowers. Others experienced the vortex of energies spiralling down into the bowl or flowing into the water as if with conscious intent.

Magic

What we are talking about here is not science as it is known today. What most essence makers and essence practitioners are doing is magic, pure and simple. Now magic is a set of processes that couldn't get more scientific if it tried, but what we are dealing with here is not the actuality but the perception, and from an orthodox scientific point of view all this is easily categorised and dismissed as psychism, self-delusion, non-validated, non-verifiable wishful thinking. No matter how essence users agree to the terminologies of resonance, vibration, chakras, subtle bodies, electromagnetic fields and other models and paradigms, to the guardians of consensus reality they are all stark staring nuts. Until, that is, someone directly experiences and benefits from the very real, potent life-changing effects that using essences can bring about. From a starting point of cynical disbelief, the newly converted essence user begins to learn the lingo, the jargon of rationalisation, and refers to energy patterns, learns about the chakras, the meridians and so on. All this puts into a justifiable consensus context an experience that is beyond understanding.

We do not know what essences really are. We do not know how they work – in terms of acceptable scientific understanding. Falling outside of science, they, of necessity, remain magical.

Definitions

There is perhaps nothing as subversive as essences – anyone can make them, they are undetectable by present technologies yet are still able to bring about significant healing and personal spiritual development for little financial outlay, using few resources, and with no adverse side effects. But, paradoxically, even the term 'essence' is very difficult to pin down, seeming to circle around any exact meaning.

'Essence' is defined by the *Oxford English Dictionary* as follows:

1. Being viewed as a fact or as a property of something.

2. Something that is; an entity. Now only as a spiritual entity.

3. Specific being 'what a thing is'; nature, character.

4. Substance: the substratum of phenomena; absolute being.

5. That by which anything subsists.

6. Essentiality.

7. That which constitutes the being of a thing, either (a) as a conceptual, or (b) as a real, entity; that by which it is what it is.

8. The specific difference of anything.

9. An extract obtained by distillation or otherwise from a plant or drug and containing its specific properties in a reduced form. In pharmacy, an alcoholic solution of the volatile elements or essential oil.

10. A perfume, a scent.

So what is an essence?

An essence is an energy signature of a plant, a place or some other focus often held in water, usually preserved in brandy or another alcohol. Orthodox testing would reveal nothing other than water and alcohol – there is no physical presence of the source at all.

The most sensitive apparatus available to us is our own body, and it is on this that the essences can have immediate and profound effects that are experienced from a subjective viewpoint.

CHAPTER 2

THE WONDER OF WATER

To begin to understand the way essences are made and are thought to work it is worth looking more closely at the carrier of most essences – water. Water covers around 71 per cent of the surface of the Earth; 98 percent of that 71 per cent is in the oceans. We are 70 per cent water. We also have other special relationships with water – too much – we die; too little – we die.

Water is a prerequisite for life to even have evolved on this planet. Enzymes and other compounds that are necessary for life do not work without water. Water is the second most common molecule in the universe, the first being hydrogen (H_2).

Although water has been widely studied, its properties continue to intrigue scientists and hints of its abilities are not completely understood by many. Most people know the chemical formula for water: H_2O. This means that for every oxygen atom, there are two hydrogen atoms.

To try to understand why water is so special the Periodic Table of Elements (see Figure 2.1) needs to be examined. It holds a lot of information about the different elements that make up our environment and how they relate to one another. This table as we see it today was built up over 150 years. Though most people attribute it to Mendeleev in 1869, it is still being adjusted today in the 21st century to accommodate new discoveries.

The table shows, at the top left is the lightest element, hydrogen (H). Following the table downwards shows the number of electrons, protons and neutrons in the atom increasing. This is reflected by the atomic number and the fact that the atoms themselves get heavier as the elements change name and quality.

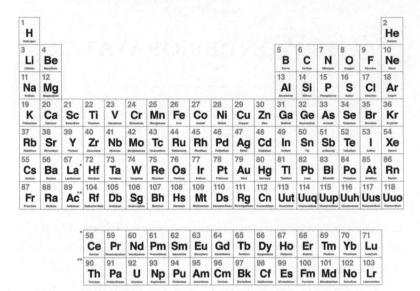

FIGURE 2.1 The Periodic Table

The table also shows what Mendeleev did and that was to arrange the elements with similar properties together. This also enabled scientists to see where there were gaps for unknown elements, like the later named germanium. For example, in the second column we have several elements that are related to one another and that are known from mineralogy – beryllium, magnesium, calcium, strontium and barium. The further down the listing, the heavier the atom is, so if a piece of gypsum/selenite (calcium sulphate) is compared with a similar sized piece of celestite, the celestite would be noticeably heavier. Celestite is strontium sulphate $SrSO_4$, and strontium is a much heavier atom than calcium.

If we look at where oxygen is in the table, top right, it is surrounded by lots of other elements (see Figure 2.2).

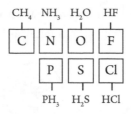

C – Carbon	CH$_4$ is Methane
N – Nitrogen	NH$_3$ is Ammonia
F – Fluorine	FH is Hydrogen Fluoride
P – Phosphorus	PH$_3$ is Phosphine
S – Sulphur	H$_2$S is Hydrogen Sulphide
Cl – Chlorine	HCl is Hydrogen Chloride or Hydrochloric acid

FIGURE 2.2 Part of the Periodic Table showing the position of oxygen

Their proximity in the Table would suggest that these elements form similar compounds that behave in a similar way. When they combine with hydrogen this is indeed the case, apart from when oxygen and hydrogen mix.

Carbon + Hydrogen	= Methane	– a gas at room temperature
Nitrogen + Hydrogen	= Ammonia	– a gas at room temperature
Fluorine + Hydrogen	= Hydrogen Fluoride	– a gas at room temperature
Phosphorus + Hydrogen	= Phosphine	– a gas at room temperature
Sulphur + Hydrogen	= Hydrogen Sulphide	– a gas at room temperature
Chlorine + Hydrogen	= Hydrogen Chloride	– a gas at room temperature

All these gases are dangerous to health and poisonous in large quantities. It should follow that the combination of oxygen with hydrogen would be a gas at room temperature and would also be poisonous – but it is neither. It breaks the rules. Water is weird!

Water molecules

One of the reasons for the weird behaviour of water is thought to be how the molecules of water interact with each other.

The water molecule is sometimes called the 'Mickey Mouse' molecule, mainly because it can be represented like this:

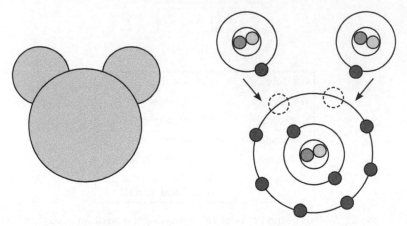

FIGURES 2.3 AND 2.4 Water: the 'Mickey Mouse' molecule

However, there is an imbalance or inequality of how the oxygen atom and hydrogen atoms share their electrons. In effect the atoms become tiny magnets and they start to attract other molecules. This phenomenon is called 'hydrogen bonding' (see Figure 2.5).

These bonds are strong enough in water to give water its unusual properties. DNA and enzymes both depend on the hydrogen bonding of water. Surface tension is also evidence of hydrogen bonding.

If there were no hydrogen bonding – there would be no life.

If there were slightly weaker bonding – life would exist at lower temperatures.

If there were slightly stronger bonding – life would exist at higher temperatures.

If the bonding were much stronger – there would be no life.

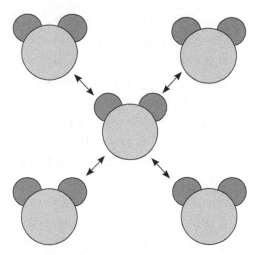

Figure 2.5 Hydrogen bonding

Hydrogen bonding in water means that at 4°C water is at its maximum density. Above that temperature its volume expands and below that its volume also expands. Water becomes crystalline (ice) at 0°C. Other compounds become denser as they get colder.

At atomic levels small clusters of water group together. This can happen in several ways and many 'types' of water have been identified. Ordinarily the clusters form and reform, some identical to others, some with similar part-patterns. This was only confirmed in 1998, but the idea of molecules replicating a pattern has been summed up by the phrase 'the memory of water', used by Jacques Benveniste (1935–2004). This brilliant man stirred up a lot of controversy over his experiments with water, which cost him his research post and some say he never recovered from the stress of those events.

His work was reported widely. Several laboratories set about reproducing his experiments and all succeeded except one, yet it was this one that was brought to everyone's notice through the media. He was subsequently labelled as a quack and fraudster.

The memory of water is very short unless other materials or substances are present. So if water has a memory that needs to be preserved some ethanol could be added. This is what Dr Edward Bach did with the Bach Flower Remedies in 1928–1936. Other preservatives are vinegar, citricidal, honey, salt and glycerol. Using spring water as a starting point helps too, as it contains minute amounts of minerals that encourage the creation of the bonding mechanism. Even using glass equipment helps because some of the ions from the glass move into the water.

Succussion, or rapid shaking of a liquid, encourages the patterns in the water to replicate, as in homoeopathic dilutions, but there is no explanation as to why a human being is then able to react and use this pattern as a healing tool.

In mineralogy, individual gems and crystals can be identified by the way the crystal lattice deflects laser light, and the angle between the atoms is so precise that correct identification can be made because the angle is always the same for that molecule.

The atomic bonding angle in water, however, is not constant (see Figure 2.6). It varies from 104.27° to 109.28°, the norm being accepted as 104.35° – this suggests that there could be lots of different 'waters', a belief held by many water energy experts.

Water Molecule

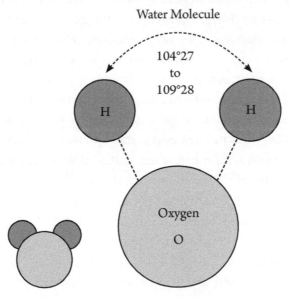

FIGURE 2.6 The atomic bonding angle in water

Dr Bernard Grad (1920–2010) of McGill University discovered in the 1960s that if water was subjected to a small magnetic field or to light, the atomic bonding in the water would be altered and there is also a reduction in surface tension. He went on to show that a person can emit enough of a magnetic field to alter the atomic bonds of water. Indeed, when someone focused positive intent into the water and that water subsequently was used to water plants it resulted in strong growth of the plants. The effect of water focused on by someone who was upset or disturbed was shown to produce little or no additional growth in plants.

More recent research, first published in English in 2005 by Professor Bernd Kröplin from the University of Stuttgart, has looked at the mechanisms by which water collects, stores and disseminates information. He showed that even the temporary influence of weak energy fields can cause changes in water structure. He also showed that the effect on the water was influenced by the experimenter, so the phenomenon cannot be reproduced independently of an observer. In effect any work on water structure cannot ever be objective. The observer is inescapably part of the experiment, and their mood adds to the effect on the water. This last sentence is very important as it may well explain some of the failures by other researchers to reproduce Jacques Benveniste's experiments in 1988.

Kröplin and his team took the work further. They looked at what happens when a single drop of water dries on a glass slide and is then observed through a dark-field lens. (The use of 'dark field' excludes the unscattered beams of light from the image. This leaves the image on a black background.) It was observed that distilled water left no trace. Different homoeopathic potencies produced different patterns, distinctly different from water. Minnie Hein, a member of the research team, was familiar with essences. She calls them 'informed' water as they have not been serially diluted and succussed. Water drops from the same essence dried by her and a colleague appeared slightly different from each other, though the basic characteristics remained the same. This also suggested that the experimenter was influencing the structure of the drops in some way. Even the same experimenter on different days using the same essence resulted in dried drops that varied slightly.

Minnie Hein came to the conclusion that the dried drop was a joint picture of experimenter and 'informed' water. Over time this experiment was repeated again and again with different people, showing slightly varied drops. Experiments continued using human saliva. Two samples were collected by several experimenters. One was collected before people anchored their personal energies to the planet (being grounded) and calmed themselves (being centred), and the second taken after they had done so. Not only were the drops more coherent after each person was grounded and centred, but the drops taken by each experimenter also had their own characteristics.

The team also looked at the dried drops of saliva when subjected to electromagnetic fields, like those produced by mobile phones. The subjected drops showed structures that were more rigid and less diverse.

Research has also been conducted by several people into how water flowing in certain ways affects the surface tension – in effect making it 'wetter'. The most well known of these researchers was Vicktor Schauberger (1855–1958). He discovered that if flowing water was made to pass through a vortex that spins the water anticlockwise towards the apex, it affected the surface tension of the water. By drinking water that has been 'spun' the body seems to heal quicker and become stronger.

Several studies have been carried out on the physical properties of homoeopathic potentised water. Wursumser (1948), Gay and Boiron (1953) and Stephenson (1955) investigated the way light is absorbed by various potencies of chemicals like sodium chloride. They showed that anomalies in the light absorption of the various potencies could be measured and plotted to reflect the dilutions. Ansaloni and Vecchi in 1989 did similar work with water that had been potentised by healers.

Water responds to sound and can produce surface wave patterns when subjected to music (Hans Jenny (1904–1972) and Alexander Lauterwasser (1951–)) The more popular work by Masaru Emoto

(1943–) has shown that ice crystals reflect the coherence of the music that the liquid was subjected to before it was frozen.

In conclusion it can be clearly seen that there has been a significant body of research into the phenomenon we call water and to how it holds energy patterns. Serial dilution and succussion has been shown to change how water reacts. The popular media and its pundits are always keen to trash homoeopathy and the 'fanciful' idea that water has memory on the premise that there is no scientific evidence, even when there is plenty of replicable work done by brave researchers who are prepared to see for themselves, refusing to be confined to what they have been taught, or by the expectations and results of their peers.

CHAPTER 3

HISTORY OF ESSENCES

Flower essences are thought to have been used by various civilisations for centuries. Among the native peoples of the world, flowers and plants are the primary source of healing and spiritual energies. The power of each plant is believed to come from its spirit. To engage with this spirit many cultures will include preparations from the required plants by making broths, baths, bundles, oils, tinctures and so on, so that they may be administered externally or internally. The chemical properties of the plant may or may not be employed in a conscious manner – the spirit is all important. We shall see too, that in modern flower essence usage, in the end, subtracting all the jargon and pseudo-scientific terminology, it also comes back to the same thing: the intangible, indefinable, immeasurable spirit of the plant.

The most equivalent technique used in Europe seems to have been the collection of morning dew off flowers and leaves recorded in medieval European magical traditions. Hildegard von Bingen (1098–1179) has been revered for her writings on plants and nature, though no authenticated copies survive confirming that she did this. Manuscripts written over a century after her death are the only copies that have been validated. Nevertheless there is no doubt she had great sensitivity to the plants available to her.

Paracelsus (1493–1541) was thought to have used dew water from flowers. He also put flowers of the plant Retamon Palermo (*Genista benehoavens*) in water and preserved the resulting liquid in schnapps. This was then used in the winter months to uplift emotions and to maintain energy. Paracelsus was primarily a synthesist of Classical and native (pagan) healing and spiritual techniques, it is reasonable to assume that he was borrowing from already established sources.

Dr Edward Bach (1886–1936) was a particularly gifted doctor and researcher. His disillusionment with some of the conventional treatments of the time drew him to look at natural sources, mainly plants, to treat the emotional states he saw as the basis of many diseases.

Dr Bach seems to have combined the magical dew-collecting of Paracelsus with the theoretical background of homoeopathy. Led by direct personal intuitive insights he began by roaming the countryside at dawn collecting and drinking the dew off certain plants. For practical reasons he developed other collecting and preparation techniques that are still in use today.

From 1928 until 1934 he created 20 flower essences made by what is now known as 'the traditional sunlight method', the same method used by Paracelsus and the Australian Aboriginals. The remaining 18 Bach Flower Remedies he made in the last 18 months of his life by boiling plant material and preserving the resulting liquid. From his death in 1936 and until 1967 these were the only flower essences widely available.

In 1967 Dr Arthur Bailey from Yorkshire created The Bailey Flower Essences. Arthur Bailey had a rigorous scientific background, but had always had a love of nature and felt particularly drawn towards flowers though healing and meditation and it was from this background that his essences were developed.

In the 1970s, Richard Katz and Patricia Kaminski developed the Californian Flower Essences prepared from plants indigenous to the United States (mainly California). Lila Devi, also from the USA, started work on 'The Master's Essences', now known as 'Spirit-in-Nature Essences', made from many familiar fruit and vegetable flowers.

Historically the next essence maker in 1985 was Ellie Web, from Galloway in southwest Scotland. Her selection of flower essences reflects the wild flowers in her surroundings. In 1990 with his curiosity aroused by the lack of a Bach Flower Remedy made from hazel, Simon Lilly began looking at the trees that had not been included in the Bach range. The result was Green Man Essences, one of the first ranges of essences in a new wave of UK essence producers that went on to blossom further in 1997, following the International Flower Essence Conference at Findhorn.

In 1997/8 Rose Titchiner, Sue Monk, Patricia Staines and Rosemary Potter began plans to hold the first essence gathering in Leiston, Suffolk with the intention of setting up an association as part of the programme. The BFVEA (British Flower and Vibrational Essences Association, www.bfvea.com) was born on 4 May 1998 at 2:52pm. It was agreed that the BFVEA would be a practitioner association with an appropriate Code of Conduct and that the BFVEA would provide a quarterly journal called *Essence* to be published on the equinoxes and solstices. At the BFVEA 1999 Gathering held at Crossmead, Exeter, the BFVEA agreed the core subjects to be taught in all BFVEA-approved essence courses.

In 1999 the situation around the legality of essence creation and the future of essences shifted with the proposal of the European Union's Traditional Herbal Medicines Directive (THMD) and it became apparent that there would need to be a special effort to keep essences safe. In the following year it was recognised that the amount of pro-active effort that was needed to protect the future of essence production and essence use in the UK would distort and weaken the broad role of the BFVEA. It was therefore agreed that a sister association, the British Association of Flower Essence Producers (BAFEP), should be formed to take over that role, allowing the BFVEA to focus its attention on practitioners and courses.

On 28 September 2000 at 2:15pm, BAFEP was inaugurated. One of its first tasks was to disseminate guidelines of production, labelling and advertising that were already part of UK law. This is made freely available to anyone enquiring about making essences and is also on the BAFEP website so it is available to government agencies. To help clarify the essence situation in the UK, a meeting with the Medicines Control Agency (MCA) was set for June 2002.

This was a most productive session as BAFEP was able to give the full picture of essence production in the UK, the breadth of which had not been appreciated by the government. Subsequently it was agreed with the Foods Standards Agency and the MCA that essences would be classed as foods. (In the UK there are only three possible categories – foods, medicines or cosmetics – each with their own guidelines restrictions and laws.) If essences had been left to fall under the auspices of the European Union Traditional Herbal Medicine Directive (THMD), a medicinal category, then virtually all essence production would have stopped. Essences would have been categorised as medicines, requiring expensive licenses for each item, laboratory-like conditions for production and scientific proof of any claims made.

Essences are still categorised by the Medicines and Health Products Regulatory Agency (MHRA, formerly the MCA) as 'borderline products' that can be marketed as foods or medicines depending on what the producer wants. If a producer decides to market their essences as medicines then licenses must be paid for, scientific proof acquired and medicinal manufacturing procedures need to be followed. If a producer wants to market their essences as foods they follow food production procedures, but do not make any medicinal claims for their essences.

The MHRA provides a list of indicative words that can be construed to show that a product is a medicine if used to describe that product (see Chapter 16). One of these words is 'remedy'. Bach Flower Remedies have been given a special exemption on historical grounds to continue to use the word 'remedy' and 'remedies'. No other essence producer has been granted this. This is the main reason that the term 'essence' tends to be used nowadays.

The MHRA stated in early 2005 that registration for the Bach Flower Remedies' range under the THMD was 'implausible'. It is thought that this was due to the inclusion in the range of essence 'Rock Water', which is not a plant. Rock Water is created by simply leaving spring water in a bowl which is left open to the sunlight. Failure to slip Bach Flower Remedies into the THMD allowed the process of essences being secured under the 'foods' category to begin.

After adjustments in Food Directives within the EC, BAFEP had another meeting with the Food Standards Agency (FSA) and MHRA in late August 2005 to ensure a safe 'home' for all essences within UK law. BAFEP were advised to carry out research to back the emotional and psychological claims for UK essences. Professor Michael E. Hyland of the University of Plymouth carried out research on the Bach Flower Remedies to meet that requirement (see Appendix 3). In addition to the research done at the University of Plymouth, BAFEP created an online, searchable database of essences that is available on the website (www.bafep.com), which catalogues essences by producer, type, making method and subtle energy map designation (chakra, element etc.). This has proved to be a fantastic resource for not only the essence practitioner but also for researchers and governmental agencies.

In 2013 the BFVEA helped to form the essence therapy lead body with The Bach Centre. The lead body is called the Confederation of Registered Essence Practitioners (COREP) and is recognised by the federal regulator – the General Regulatory Council for Complementary Therapies (GRCCT). The legacy of Dr Edward Bach is alive and well.

In 2014 there were over 150 essence producers in the UK, over 50 of whom belong to the British Association of Flower Essence Producers (BAFEP). The UK has more essence producers than the rest of the world put together!

CHAPTER 4

TYPES OF ESSENCES

Many people are unaware that even within the Bach Flower range there are two types of essence – 37 flower and plant essences and one environmental essence. Since the early 1970s many other types of essence have become available and many ways of creating essences have been discovered.

In 1998/9 the use of essences in Brazil was threatened by moves to stop doctors from using any alternative practices that were not scientifically approved. Quickly following this, some pharmacists who were providing dosage bottles of flower essences were threatened by consumer rights officials. Essences are used widely in Brazil, and can often be the only help available when there is a lack of finances. A group of essence users, including Ruth Toledo Altshuler, got together to create a classification framework for the Brazilian government. In doing so they created a comprehensive list of the types of essences available. As a result of their hard work, essences continue to be widely used in Brazil. Nowadays there are postgraduate courses in essence use, and essences are used in hospitals and in many research programmes and clinical trials.

The list which follows is based on the definitions developed by Ruth Toledo Altschuler and her colleagues. (Details about the methods of making essences can be found in Chapter 14 and Appendix 1.)

1. Flower essences

These are essences prepared from the flowers of plants. There are various methods of making these essences:

- using water/sunlight
- using water/moonlight
- using a mediator (i.e. a crystal, plant spirit)
- using a boiling method
- pouring water over flowers
- dipping live flowers into water
- using specific patterns of flowers or numbers of flowers to add another focus of shape or number
- indirect methods.

The flowers of a plant are the primary visual communicators of a plant. They attract pollinators and their colours and shapes attract appreciation from humans. Essences made from flowers continue this function of mutual relationship and sharing with the greater world.

2. Plant essences

These are essences that are prepared from the fruit, root, stem, twig or seed of a plant:

- using sunlight/water
- using moonlight/water
- using a boiling method
- using a mediator (i.e. a crystal, plant spirit)
- indirect methods.

Different parts of a plant have different biological functions: for example, the leaves help with respiration, roots draw nutrients from the soil and seeds are the means of reproduction. The function of a particular part of a plant will be reflected in the essence made from that part.

3. Mineral, crystal or gem essences

These are essences that are prepared from minerals, crystal and gems. When prepared without preservatives these are usually referred to as 'gem waters'. Care must be taken with minerals, crystals and gems as some are poisonous. They are made:

- using sunlight/water

- using moonlight/water

- using patterns or specific numbers of minerals, crystals or gems to add another focus

- indirect methods.

Minerals and crystals are precise and coherent energy patterns. Essences made from minerals and crystals help to create harmony in every level.

4. Environmental vibrational essences

This type of essence is very popular and is growing fast. An essence is made of a landscape, sacred site or during a specific natural event:

- using sunlight/water

- using moonlight/water

- using a mediator (i.e. a crystal)

- using specific astronomical or astrological timing.

Environmental essences allow access to their particular qualities by anybody, anywhere, anytime.

4b. *Channelled essences*

This is another method that is very popular. Here the essence producer invites a specific energy or entity to co-create an essence:

- using a focus to channel the energies

- a mediator is used (such as a spirit guide etc.).

This type of essence is dependent on the clarity of the producer and their ability to link into the target of the essence. Essences made this way allow anyone to have access to the focus of the essence.

5. Radionic/energy essences

These methods introduce patterns to water using energy devices and thereby delivering them in a traditional way or using digital means, like MP3 audio files:

- using devices like pendulums, radionics equipment like the 'Black box', computer programs, energy rings, etc.

Digital means of delivering essences are beginning to grow in popularity. The focus of the essences can be anything that the producer feels is appropriate.

6. General essences

These are essences that do not fit into any of the other categories, e.g.

- created using light/coloured light

- created using sound

- created using shapes, symbols

- essences carried by video or film.

Both sound and light/coloured light essences are very precise wavelengths of the electromagnetic spectrum and can have an immediate effect on the multilayers (the physical and subtle layers of the body) of the body.

In addition to the original list, the following can be added:

7. Composite essences

These are essences which have several components but that are made by one method at the same time. These essences tend to reflect the harmony, unity and relationship that the synergistic method produces.

8. Combination essences

These essences have several individual components that may be different types of essence or essences made at different times of the year brought together to create a combination for a specific reason – for example, first-aid combinations.

If it is the signature of the entire plant that becomes integrated into the structure of the water, then why are the flowers the parts so often used? It is true that nowadays essences are being made from all parts of plants from root to seed and all are effective. It may be that there are slightly different emphases to an essence made from a root, a leaf, a seed. In general, it is the flower that is most commonly used to make an essence. If we think of our appreciation – where our attention travels to – whole businesses are built on this attraction to the shape, colour and smell of flowers. Of all the parts of a plant, the flower is the most specifically created to interact with its environment: the flower is the communication vehicle of a plant. It is there to be noticed, to be smelled, to be crawled into, to be sucked, to be pollinated by something of another realm – be that insect, bird, animal or the wind and rain. The peculiar structure of each flower acknowledges the many mechanisms of the outer world, the 'not-I'. It is this interaction with the 'not-I' upon which the continuation of the plants and its species ultimately depends. This outwards expression of the life-force of the plants is thus perceived by us as being the powerful culmination of growth, of manifestation, of individuality, of self-awareness. Our emotions are almost automatically and immediately affected by colour, smell and shape of a flower in a way that a leaf or stem fails to achieve. The immediate appreciation of a flower that we as humans feel, the aesthetic of the sense perceptions, shows us a biological reality. Flowers are biologically important for our survival.

The flower is like a psychic head, eye, voice and message drawing our attention and holding us in focused but free-floating contemplation. With such a deep-felt contact carefully picking a few flower heads, placing them on water and treating them as reverential offerings from another Kingdom – the message and the messenger – is a natural ritual interaction.

Excerpt from *Tree: Essence of Healing*, Simon and Sue Lilly, 1999.

CHAPTER 5

Selecting Essences

Essences and homoeopathy have always had very close links. It comes as no great surprise therefore that the most familiar selection of essences requires the practitioner to know what each essence is said to be used for and to match the issues of the client to the properties of the most appropriate essence.

It has been recognised, however, that this process can have its limitations and there are many other methods for choosing essences that are appropriate for personal use or working with other people. There are actually no hard and fast rules to any of these methods, though each method has its advantages and disadvantages.

Logic and pattern-matching

This is a technique frequently used by homoeopaths and many Bach Flower Remedy practitioners. In this method the practitioner listens to the client as they describe how they feel and what they think. The practitioner then uses their knowledge of the essences they have available to them to match the emotional and mental pattern of the client with the descriptions given for the essences. The advantages of this technique are:

- It can be used by anyone.

- It is already familiar to clients as it is used by orthodox health professionals and some complementary and alternative health professionals.

- It encourages practitioners to study and read as much as they can about the essences they use.

- Any selection can be tailored to a specific need or outcome.

- The practitioner can show the client what has been written about each essence choice confirming reasoning behind the suggested essence(s).

The disadvantages of this technique are:

- The practitioner is dependent on what the client presents (appearance, tone of voice, verbal description of feelings, thoughts and symptoms etc.).

- It relies on what a producer or author has described about what they think an essence's qualities are.

- It can be dependent on the listening, questioning and counselling skills of the practitioner to get a full and accurate picture of the client's situation.

Dowsing

This is a technique where the practitioner dowses, usually with a pendulum, over the selection of essences they have to hand to determine the most effective essence(s) for the client. Sometimes a practitioner will dowse from a list or an arc showing the essences they have available. The advantages of this technique are:

- The technique is easy to learn.

- The practitioner is not totally dependent on what the client is able to verbalise.

- The practitioner does not have to have detailed intellectual knowledge of the essences they have available.

- Selection of the appropriate essence(s) is quick.

- Selection can be focused on a specific client need.

The disadvantages of this technique are:

- It is dependent for accuracy on the ability of the practitioner to remain grounded, detached and to have no expectations as to the resultant choices.

- If the practitioner does not explain what they are doing the client can feel left out of the process.

- Some clients may be wary of a practitioner using a pendulum.

- It is possible for either the practitioner or client or both to affect the pendulum response.

Muscle testing

Muscle testing was originally developed by George Goodheart. Muscle testing is based on the concepts of Traditional Chinese Medicine and the meridian system and is seen as a non-invasive way of evaluating the body's imbalances and assessing its needs.

The practitioner assesses the client's ability to maintain the position of one of their muscles, with the minimum of effort, when subject to the application of gentle pressure by the practitioner.

A muscle is chosen, usually in the arm, and when properly set the resilience of this muscle will indicate the energy flow in the body of the client. The advantages of this technique are:

- It involves the client directly in the process.

- The practitioner is not totally dependent on what the client is able to verbalise.

- The practitioner does not have to have detailed intellectual knowledge of the essences they have available.

- It is quick and flexible.

- It is less easy for the practitioner to influence the outcome compared to dowsing.

- Selection can be qualified for a specific client need.

The disadvantages of this technique are:

- It takes time for the practitioner to become confident in the technique.

- It can be difficult to use on clients who train with weights in a gym as their muscles are less responsive to small changes within their bodies.

- It can be difficult to use with clients on pharmaceutical drugs, especially those used to treat emotions or moods as these drugs can have a disruptive effect on the meridian system.

- Some clients may be wary of a practitioner using muscle testing.

Self-testing or finger testing

Self-testing or finger testing is similar to dowsing but here the practitioner uses their own muscles responses (usually the hands/ fingers) to determine choices. The advantages of this technique are:

- The technique is easy to learn.

- The practitioner is not totally dependent on what the client is able to verbalise.

- The practitioner does not have to have detailed intellectual knowledge of the essences they have available.

- Selection of the appropriate essence(s) is quick.

- Selection can be qualified for a specific client need.

The disadvantages of this technique are:

- It is dependent for accuracy on the ability of the practitioner to remain grounded, detached and have no expectation of the outcome.

- Some clients may be wary of a practitioner using a self-testing technique.

- If the practitioner does not explain what they are doing, the client can feel left out or confused by the process.

Client preference

This is a technique where the client is asked a series of questions – for example, what their favourite plant/tree/colour/weather is, and then what they dislike. Both can be indicative of the client's needs. The 'like' can show what the client is attracted to that maintains their sense of well-being. The 'dislike' can show what the client is avoiding and can indicate what the subconscious or unconscious needs are to redress any imbalances. The practitioner then translates this to correlate with the essences. The advantages of this technique are:

- It involves the client directly.

- It can shed light on some of the deeper needs of the client.

- The practitioner is not totally dependent on what the client is able to verbalise.

- The practitioner does not have to have detailed intellectual knowledge of the essences they have available.

- Selection of the appropriate essence(s) is quick.

- Selection can be qualified for a specific client need, depending on the questions asked by the practitioner.

The disadvantages of this technique are:

- The practitioner needs to know their essences in depth.

- The practitioner can be limited or restricted to the choices made by the client.

- The client may be reticent about trusting the outcome.

Intuition

This is a technique where the practitioner is instructed by their inner guidance to what would be the most effective essence(s). The advantages of this technique are:

- Everyone can do it.

- The practitioner is not totally dependent on what the client is able to verbalise.

- The practitioner does not have to have detailed intellectual knowledge of the essences they have available.

- Selection of the appropriate essence(s) is quick.

- Selection can be qualified for a specific client need.

The disadvantages of this technique are:

- It can take time for the practitioner to become confident.

- It is dependent for accuracy on the ability of the practitioner to remain grounded, detached and have no expectations of the outcome.

- The practitioner may be over-confident, may have very rigid ideas that limit their perspective or may feel pressure to impress others with their skills.

- If the practitioner does not explain what they are doing, the client can feel left out of the process.

- Some clients may be wary of a practitioner using their intuition.

Visual images

Nowadays many essence ranges have sets of photographs or symbols linked to each essence. These can be shown to the client for them to choose what they like or what they think they need as well as what they dislike. The 'like' can show what the client is attracted to that maintains their sense of well-being. The 'dislike' can show what the client is avoiding and can indicate what the subconscious or unconscious needs to redress any imbalances. The advantages of this technique are:

- Everyone can do it.

- The practitioner is not totally dependent on what the client is able to verbalise.

- The practitioner does not have to have detailed intellectual knowledge of the essences they have available.

- With symbols the client is less likely to be influenced by conscious preferences.

- Selection of the appropriate essence(s) is quick.

- Selection can be qualified for a specific client need.

The disadvantages of this method are:

- With photographs the client may avoid selecting images that are less pretty or attractive.

- The client may doubt the significance of their choices and not have much confidence in the outcome.

Other factors in selection of essences

In most cases it can be helpful for the practitioner to have an idea of what outcome is desired. It helps to focus any of the above selection techniques. It is always a welcome change to be asked to help someone with an aspirational goal, rather than 'fixing' an issue.

Here are some examples of the possible areas, goals or problems that can the choice of essences can focus on (there may be more than one focus):

1. Physical – a physical problem where the underlying emotional and mental stresses might be helped by the use of essences.

2. Emotional – an emotional problem that essences might help to release.

3. Mental – a mental attitude, belief or psychological problem that essences might help to ease.

4. Spiritual – a spiritual or philosophical problem that essences might help to unravel.

5. Subtle – when there is some evidence of subtle energy imbalance or disturbance (meridian, chakra or subtle body) within the client's description of their problems.

6. Constitutional (as in the homoeopathic sense) – a particular essence that will always help the person, regardless of what the problem is.

7. Underlying life theme – an essence(s) to help with developing personal potential, help with finding personal direction or help with releasing karma.

8. Underlying family theme – an essence(s) to help to release problems around a theme or pattern within the family that needs to be addressed.

9. An immediate issue – an essence(s) to help with the stress and build-up of a driving test next week or a forthcoming interview or exam.

10. As a key to other issues – an essence(s) that will act as a key to help find what the underlying problem really is.

11. Current issue only – an essence(s) for emergency use, short-term use.

12. Supportive, but not specific to the current situation – an essence(s) to act as ongoing support.

13. Needed cyclically – monthly, yearly, two-yearly, seven-yearly, etc. – an essence(s) to help deal with an anniversary pattern or an astrological pattern.

14. Anchoring an issue to a place (where the essence(s) was made) or a time (when the essence(s) was made – day, year, season, moon phase, etc.).

15. Links to a specific producer – themselves personally, their approach, how they make their essences.

16. Plant Spirit Teacher – an essence that links to a plant that could be a personal guide for healing and learning.

17. Anything else?

(It is also a good idea to have an 'anything else?' option in case there is something that has not been immediately obvious.)

How many essences in one 'go'?

A single essence may not be appropriate to help deal with issues of a particular client. Many practitioners make up 'dosage' bottles for their clients from the stock bottles provided by producers. Before doing that it is a good idea to check with producers what dilution level they provide. Dilutions labelled 5× or 1:100,000 are already at the 'dosage' level.

There are no 'rules' as to how many drops or how many different essences can be put into a personal dosage combination. However, bear in mind that each essence is a specific vibration so there will a limit to how much vibrational information the client's body will be able to process. Provide too much information and the client's body may ignore it all. Sometimes less is better!

If someone is already taking pharmaceutical drugs or homoeopathic help, essences are unlikely to affect either. However, taking essences may reduce the body's need for the dosage of pharmaceuticals prescribed by a medical professional. Alternately if a client is very unwell or has low levels of prana (life-force) in their body, they will be unable to process a lot of energy information, so may be overwhelmed in conjunction with homoeopathic treatment.

Even with the presence of pharmaceuticals or homoeopathics, a person's body may prefer a small amount of input, so even a single essence at one drop per use might be needed to ensure that the body does not become overwhelmed.

It is usually accepted that one to six essences are placed into a personal dosage combination, but again, there are no hard-and-fast rules. The key is to provide what is appropriate.

CHAPTER 6

ASSESSMENT SKILLS

This chapter covers the use of dowsing or kinesiology (muscle testing) to assess requirements of the client. These are the primary practical tools of the complementary and alternative practitioner.

Detailed, in-depth knowledge of essences is not required to the same extent for the logic/knowledge methods of assessment if the optimal requirements of the client can be pinpointed using kinesiology or dowsing.

Care needs to be taken using either of these methods to ensure that the beliefs and predilections of the practitioner doing the assessment do not interfere with the results. There are many ways of doing this. A technique called 'tapping in', described below, is one of the simplest that can be used whenever any form of energy or healing work is done. It not only protects from surrounding energies, but also helps to ensure that the interference of personal beliefs is kept to a minimum.

'Tapping in'

The core of this technique is the tapping of the fingertips around the thymus area (top of chest). This brings into balance all the major energy meridians of the body for about 20 minutes (see Figure 6.1).

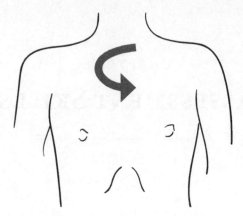

FIGURE 6.1 The thymus area

1. The simplest variation is a firm, light tapping with the fingertips on the area of the upper chest just below where the collarbones (clavicles) meet the breast bone (sternum). This is the approximate placement of the thymus gland, which is an important maintainer of the subtle energy balance in the body.

2. Whilst the thymus is being tapped, the other hand is placed palm open, over the navel. This allows the balancing effect to be longer lasting.

3. Another variation of 'tapping in' is to tap anticlockwise (if one is looking down onto the chest) in a circle about 8–15 cm away from the thymus point. Each tap of the fingers should be about 3 cm apart. Repeat the circle about 20 times.

4. Many important meridian channels pass close to the navel. Tapping around the navel about 8–10 cm away, this time in a clockwise direction, also has a balancing and centring effect.

Dowsing with a pendulum

Prior to dowsing it is important to establish a firm personal energy foundation using 'tapping in'. If personal energies are disparate, then responses from a pendulum will tend to be unreliable.

Many people have reservations about dowsing, suspecting that the pendulum can be influenced by the user. *People CAN affect the movement of a pendulum that you or someone else is using.* This is why a base line of stabilised energy needs to be created before doing any dowsing.

The pendulum represents an extension of the inner senses and amplifying and creating a visual representation of inner energy changes as they occur. The swing of the pendulum is a reaction to small muscle movements that are caused by these energy changes. The user and others can therefore influence its movement if there are strong emotional issues at play. This tendency can be effectively reduced by 'tapping in' and by maintaining a level of open curiosity in the mind.

Dowsing when somebody is emotionally charged or when there is personal investment in the answer may not be reliable.

New to dowsing?

1. If there is no bought pendulum to hand, construct a pendulum of some sort to start with – a bead on a thread is fine.

2. It is probably best in the beginning not to use personal jewellery, as it can be heavily imbued with the owner's energies.

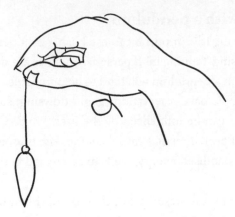

FIGURE 6.2 The dowsing pendulum

3. Holding the pendulum thread between the thumb and forefinger, with the arm bent and wrist relaxed, carry out the following exercises over the image under each paragraph:

   a. Over the straight arrow, deliberately set the pendulum in motion in a straight line away from the body. Allow it to swing back and forth for about six to eight times to get used to the feel. Stop the pendulum with the free hand.

FIGURE 6.3 Dowsing: the straight arrow

   b. Over the clockwise arrow, deliberately set the pendulum in motion in a straight line (like in exercise a), but after six to eight swings allow (intend, think it, mentally suggest, ask…) the pendulum swing to develop into a clockwise, circular or elliptic motion for six to eight rotations. Stop the pendulum with the free hand.

FIGURE 6.4 Dowsing: the clockwise arrow

c.   Over the anticlockwise arrow below, deliberately set the pendulum in motion in a straight line (like in Exercise a) but after six to eight swings allow (intend, think it, mentally suggest, ask …) the pendulum swing to develop into an anticlockwise, circular or elliptic motion for six to eight rotations. Stop the pendulum with the free hand.

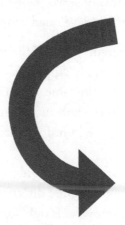

FIGURE 6.5 Dowsing: the anticlockwise arrow

d.   When confident with exercises a–c, instead of stopping the pendulum with the free hand, try stopping the pendulum by mental request or intention.

All these exercises can help to gain familiarity with the pendulum movement and to appreciate how easily anything can influence the pendulum swings.

Next step

1. 'Tap in', using the technique described earlier.

2. With the free hand placed over the solar plexus (between bottom of ribcage and navel), set the pendulum in motion on a straight-line swing.

3. Without looking at the pendulum and with an unfocused gaze, ask to be shown a 'Yes' response.

4. After 5–10 seconds, observe the pendulum and record the type of swing that has developed. Stop the pendulum.

5. Repeat 2, and ask to be shown a 'No' response.

6. After 5–10 seconds, observe the pendulum and record the type of swing that has developed. Stop the pendulum.

If the responses are different – fine. If the responses are the same, repeat the procedure after again 'tapping in'.

If the responses are still the same, leave the exercise for now and return to it another day. This whole process may need to be repeated each time dowsing is required until you have confidence with the responses.

Yes/No responses are very individual – some people have circular swings, some elliptic, some directional straight lines. Each individual needs to discover what is right for themselves.

Using lists

Lists are very useful when dowsing where a large choice of items is available. The free hand can span several lines to isolate each part of the list being assessed. Always start off with a large span for choice and then narrow the choice down into smaller numbers of lines on the list. (If 'Yes/No' is checked with every item on the list, it will take a long time and can be very tiring!) When the options are down to four or five, then they can be assessed singly.

New to self-testing or finger testing?

If information is being queried that has a high emotional personal content, these techniques may not be reliable.

It is suggested that these methods are practised until they become 'programmed' with the yes/no responses. After that, it is just practice and confidence that make these an accurate means of assessment.

Method 1

1. Tap in.

2. The left hand – allow the tips of both thumb and little finger to touch.

3. Insert the thumb and forefinger of the right hand (tips touching) into the gap between the palm of the left hand and the thumb and little finger of the left hand.

4. By parting the thumb and forefinger of the right hand forcibly outwards to contact the thumb and little finger of the left hand, the muscles holding the left-hand fingertips together are challenged.

5. If the fingertips of the left hand stay in contact or move slightly and then lock, the energy is still flowing through the muscles and for most people this indicates a 'yes' response.

6. If the fingertips of the left hand part appreciably, the muscles have weakened, and for most people this is a 'no' response.

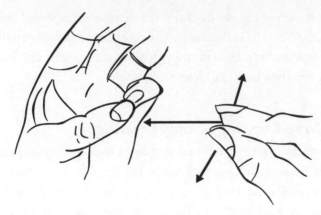

FIGURE 6.6 Finger testing: method 1

Method 2

1. Tap in.

2. Using one hand only, gently rub the thumb against the tops of the first and second finger-tips (as in the common hand gesture indicating money).

3. Whilst saying 'yes' or when a 'yes response' is indicated, the feel should be smooth.

4. Whilst saying 'no' or when indicating a 'no response' there should be more resistance.

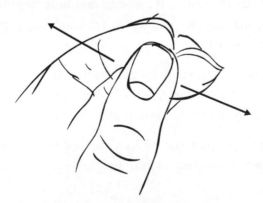

FIGURE 6.7 Finger testing: method 2

Method 3

1. Tap in.

2. On each hand, gently touch the thumb and forefinger tips.

3. Interlock each, forming a three-dimensional figure of eight.

4. Whilst saying 'yes' or when a 'yes response' is indicated, a quick movement to pull the hands apart should result in the fingertips staying in touch.

5. Whilst saying 'no' or when a 'no response' is indicated, a quick movement to pull the hands apart should be successful.

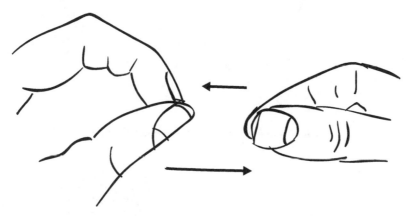

FIGURE 6.8 Finger testing: method 3

New to kinesiology (muscle testing)?

This skill takes longer to become confident with compared to dowsing.

Basic muscle testing procedure

1. Decide which muscle is going to be used.

The most commonly used in therapy situations are the brachialis variations. These can be also used in 'talking therapies' or can be used with the client lying on a couch.

The brachialis is a muscle that controls the raising and lowering of the lower arm when the elbow is supported by a couch or table. The client's hand can be either relaxed (Figure 6.9) or held with fingers out-stretched in line with the lower arm (Figure 6.10).

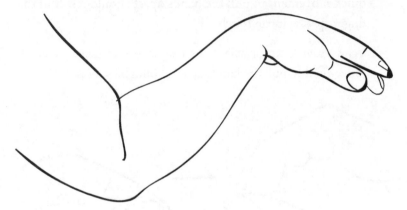

FIGURE 6.9 Muscle testing: the relaxed hand

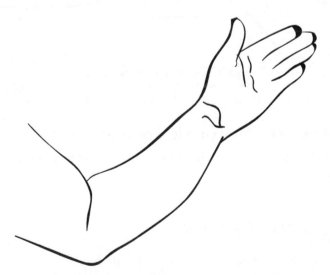

FIGURE 6.10 Muscle testing: the outstretched hand

2. The tester then gently places their flattened hand on the forearm of the client, away from the client's wrist.

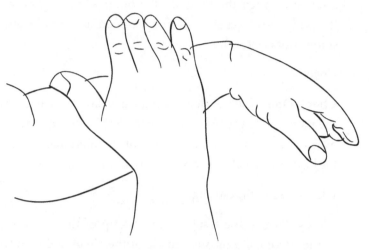

Figure 6.11 Muscle testing: tester's hand on forearm

The tester then asks the client to 'hold' their upper arm muscle firm whilst the tester slowly, evenly and gently pushes down on the client's forearm. The tester should then detect a position where his or her pushing down and the client's 'holding' are matched. This helps to determine how that muscle 'feels'. It is important to remember that this is not a muscle competition! However, it does show the interface between the tester and the client's energy.

If the client is holding the muscle too strongly, the tester should ask the client to relax their 'hold' a little or until the tester can feel some flexibility or play in the movement of the arm.

It is worth doing a few practices so that the tester and the client can be more confident about how much movement is required.

This should be a very delicate procedure. The pressure used is probably best described as the same amount needed when pushing fingers into a partly deflated balloon until you can feel the balloon tighten under the fingertips.

3. When the tester is satisfied that the muscle will work as an indicator (technically known as a SIM – strong indicator

muscle), the tester can carry out some pre-checks for something known as 'switching' (i.e. whether the energy is flowing through the body as it should; 'switching' is when the body responses show contrary or confused results due to some stress factors).

4. Checks:

Check One – ask the client to put the palm of one hand over the navel while the tester checks the SIM. (Placing the palm over the navel accesses the whole of the meridian system of the body as the palm covers sensitive points around the navel.)

If the muscle stays strong:

Check Two – The tester places the tip of the index finger of their free hand on any muscle of the client and then tests the SIM. It should weaken or lose strength. (Each fingertip acts like a pole of a magnet. Touching with a single finger creates a small electromagnetic disruption to the body.) This is repeated with the tester touching any muscle of the client with the tips of the first two fingers of the free hand – the SIM should stay strong. (Using two adjacent fingertips neutralises the electromagnetic stress because adjacent fingertips have opposite magnetic poles that cancel each other out.) This is a 'body-electric' test.

If the muscle reacts correctly:

Check Three – The tester lightly pinches the belly of any muscle of the client – the SIM should weaken or lose strength. (This test explores the nature of spindle cells and the Golgi mechanism. It is a physiological test.) The tester then smoothly massages the belly of the client's muscle and the SIM should stay strong.

If the muscle reacts correctly:

Check Four – either silently or out aloud the tester says 'Yes' whilst checking the SIM – the muscle should stay strong.

Either silently or out aloud, the tester says: 'No' whilst checking the SIM, the muscle should weaken or lose strength.

('Yes' and 'No' are straightforward childhood-based emotional responses, 'Yes' is good, positive, and 'No' is bad, negative. This is an emotional level test.)

If the SIM reacts correctly, the muscle being tested is ready to be used in assessment. If the SIM does not react as it should in any of the pre-checks, the tester needs to tap the client 'in' again and then repeat all of the checks. Once a reliable SIM has been created between the tester and the client, it can be used in a variety of ways.

Using dowsing, self-testing or kinesiology (muscle testing)

The applications of these types of assessment have no limits when dealing with essences. It is important to detach any emotions or belief from the potential outcome by 'tapping in' before starting.

Developing a good questioning technique is the most important skill after mastering the dowsing or muscle testing itself. It is almost like having to deal with a computer, there are only two answers – 'Yes' or 'No' (though with a lot of experience a 'sort of' response can be identified!)

It is important to only ask one question at a time. The body's bio-computer is very literal and some mistakes can be made if care is not taken.

Always start with broad categories – like 'Are one or more essences needed for this person?' If the indication is 'yes', then the next question could be: 'Are they from X's range?' In this way the requirements are gradually pinpointed.

When using a list start with a wide span of the hand for choice and then narrow the choice down into smaller numbers of lines on the list. Checking 'Yes/No' on every item will take a long time and can be very tiring, especially if muscle testing. When the options are down to four or five, then they can be assessed singly. Lists of essences that are available are very useful.

CHAPTER 7

USING ESSENCES

Prior to the 1990s the main way that people used essences was to take them by mouth. In the intervening years it was gradually recognised that essences were not simply liquids in bottles, they were direct energy connections to the source from which the essence was made. This has led to investigation into other ways of delivering an essence and the realisation that some methods are often more effective than taking by mouth.

By mouth

People are most familiar with essences in liquid form, either in an alcohol base or a non-alcoholic mixture, like glycerol, citricidal (grapefruit seed extract) or vinegar. Essences in these forms are easy to use 'by mouth', where a few drops are placed under the tongue or in a small glass of water to be drunk.

The advantage of using essences this way is that it is familiar to most people and reflects the common concept that essences are a sort of 'medicine'. This they are, in the broadest definition of the word. However, essences are not 'medicines' in the view of the government product regulators.

The disadvantage of this method is that it reinforces the popular idea of 'medicine' as something that is used to fix a symptom. Essences do indeed 'fix' things, but they can also do much more than that by helping the body to eliminate underlying energy imbalances. The preservative that the essence is carried in is an issue to some people. Alcohol may be unsuitable for dietary, religious or legal reasons. Glycerol, when it is used as a carrier for the essence, can act as a lubricant on the seals and stoppers of the bottles causing leaks and potential microbial contamination. Citricidal, which is a grapefruit seed extract, can be contraindicated for those taking heart medications and can also have an adverse effect on the liver and gallbladder in some people. Vinegar, depending on the type of vinegar that is used, can be unpalatable and have a persistent taste. Red shizo has been used in conjunction with vinegar, but the plant itself is a powerful herb used in Traditional Chinese Medicine, so has qualities of its own that may overwhelm the essence. The use of salt as a preservative is an easy option over alcohol, but has the disadvantages of the unpleasant taste and stress on the body from the extra salt. However, it does have the advantage that the body seems to respond to the essence much faster.

Essences can also be presented in non-alcoholic form as sugar pilules or dragees that have been soaked in the essence. The advantage of this method is that it is suitable for those who are not able to use essences in alcohol solution. Pilules or dragees can be used by children and those whose religion or beliefs prohibit the intake of alcohol. It is also easier to transport essences from country to country in pilule form. The disadvantage of this method is that it limits the use of essences to being taken by mouth.

Specific energy points

A drop of liquid essence can be placed on one or more pulse points (wrists, throat, neck, forehead, soles of the feet) or on chakras or meridian points. The semi-permeable membrane of the skin will absorb the essence quickly. Placed on the clothes the essence will affect the aura of the body. Either way, the essence will quickly have an effect on the body's energy. A drop of an essence can be put onto a tissue or cotton pad to be placed onto the point.

The advantages of this method are that the body reacts very quickly to the essence and very little essence needs to be used.

The disadvantages of this method are that clients are not familiar with the method and may be doubtful of its efficacy. If the essence is held in brandy or vinegar, then there can be a noticeable smell of the preservative present. Vodka and citricidal have little or no smell. This method cannot easily be used for essences held in glycerol as it can leave a sticky residue.

Sequential processing

Sequential processing can be quite a powerful technique to bring about rapid change in a client's situation. It is excellent for breaking down blocks, barriers and for use in emergencies.

First, the number of essences needed for the process has to be determined for the particular circumstances. Then, those essences need to be identified, as well as the order they are to be applied. There may be a repetition of some of the essences in the sequence. These requirements can be determined by logic, intuition, dowsing or muscle testing.

The process begins by placing a drop of the first essence onto the wrists of the client and then asking the client to gently rub their wrists together.

Wait about a minute, and then place the second essence of the sequence onto the wrists of the client and ask the client to rub their wrists together. This sequence is continued until the end of the determined sequence.

The advantage of this method is that it involves the client directly and the process is done in the presence of both practitioner and client.

The disadvantages of this method are that it can take a while to set up and the client may not be familiar with this method and may doubt its efficacy.

Through the aura

A few drops of the essence are placed in the palms of the hands. The palms are rubbed together and quickly swept through the energy field of the body (the aura) a few centimetres above the skin or clothes.

The advantages of this method are that the essence is activated very quickly and very little essence needs to be used. This can also be done with specific hand and sweeping movements that can link to the meridian or chakra systems.

The disadvantages of this method are that it is very obvious to an onlooker. Clients may not be familiar with the method and may be shy about using it or may doubt its efficacy.

Breathing in the essence

A few drops of the essence are placed in the palms of the hands. The palms are then rubbed together and then the hands are cupped around the nose. The evaporating essence is breathed in.

The advantages of this method are that it is probably the fastest way to introduce an essence to the body and very little essence needs to be used. It can be a discreet way of using an essence.

The disadvantages of this method are that clients may not be familiar with the method and may doubt its efficacy. The client may find the smell of the preservative off-putting or unpleasant.

Sprays

Pre-prepared essence sprays can be bought from many producers. Alternatively, a few drops of an essence can be put into a small atomiser with water.

The advantages of this method are that the spray introduces the essence to a larger area. Sprays can be used personally or they can be used for a group of people, for a room or a space. It is a quick way of introducing an essence.

The disadvantage of this method is that where the essence reaches cannot be controlled.

Carried in cosmetics

Essences can be placed in creams, lotions or massage oils.

The advantages of this method are that small amounts can be easily delivered to the body over a long period. The products are pleasant to use and can be adjusted to suit the client. It is suitable for those who are not able to use essences in alcohol solution and is easy to transport from country to country.

The disadvantages of this method are that the producer must create them under 'cosmetic law' and the testing required may increase the price for the client. Other ingredients in the product – for example, the presence of an essential oil – may compromise the efficacy of the essence. Clients may be unfamiliar with this method and doubt its efficacy.

Added to bathwater

A few drops of essence can be added to bathwater.

The advantages of this method are that it is a relaxing way to encounter the essence. The essence is absorbed through the skin and vaporised in steam.

The disadvantages of this method are that many people only use showers, so the option is not open to everyone. Clients may not like the smell of the preservative or may not be familiar with the method and may doubt its efficacy.

Images

Photographs of the item or place from which the essence was made will carry the energy of the item or place. Cards created from these can be carried, meditated upon or placed in a room to introduce the essence to the client. Symbols and shapes representing the item or place from which the essence was made can also work effectively, but in a more subtle way. Essences have also been created as short films or videos.

The advantages of this method are that most people's senses are visually dominant so it is an easy method to use. It is suitable for those who are not able to use essences in alcohol solution and easy to transport from country to country.

The disadvantage of this method is that clients may be unfamiliar with this method and doubt its efficacy.

Auditory

Essences as sounds, both obvious and subliminal, can be very useful. This method of creating an essence takes a certain amount of skill to do well.

The advantages of this method are that it can be used with subtlety. It can be used for a large space or with a group of people. It is also suitable for those who are not able to use essences in alcohol solution and easy to transport from country to country.

The disadvantages of this method are that unless the sounds are heard on headphones the area that the essence reaches cannot be controlled. Clients may be unfamiliar with this method and doubt its efficacy.

How often should essences be used?

A good guideline for using essences is three or four times a day, but it will depend on how the essence is being used. The optimal frequency, as well as the method of delivery, can be determined by dowsing or muscle testing.

How long should an essence be used for?

In some respects, if the essence is thought of as a 'key' – once the 'key' has been activated there is no need to continue to use it.

However, people's bodies and energy systems often have a level of stubbornness present with a reluctance to change. Often, there is an urge to return back to old, familiar patterns. Hence, essences may need to be used for a number of days or weeks. The ideal length of time can be determined by dowsing or muscle testing.

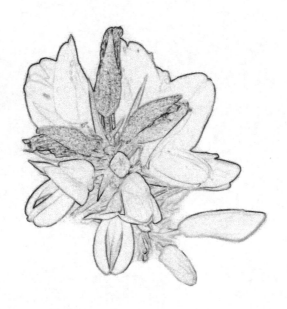

PART TWO

BACKGROUND INFORMATION TO CHOOSE AND USE ESSENCES MORE EFFECTIVELY

Background information

The next four chapters cover background information about subtle energies and subtle anatomy. Knowledge of these can bring greater understanding to the underlying processes of clients' issues, problems and aspirations. They also underpin many new ways of using essences. They can also be very useful shorthand for making notes, for understanding any essence and for discerning new essences.

CHAPTER 8

CHAKRAS

Over the last 3000 years, sages, philosophers and mystics have described the subtle energies in our environment and within our bodies in many different ways. Several systems have developed from different philosophical backgrounds. A common understanding is that wherever dynamic energies meet together in nature they form spinning circular patterns, or vortices. The Vedic seers of ancient India also perceived similar energy vortices within the energy of the human body. Wherever two or more channels of subtle energy met, there was a vortex, which they named 'chakra', meaning wheel.

Where major energy flows coincided on the midline of the body in the front of the spinal column, there the seers of India saw seven main chakras that seemed to mirror both health and spiritual well-being. These seven chakras were like multi-dimensional gateways that would allow the individual to access different experiences and states of consciousness. The use of visualisation, sound, chant, meditation and exercise to activate, cleanse and integrate these seven chakras became an important part of spiritual practice especially in the Himalayan regions of India, Nepal and Tibet.

Many of the original Vedic texts discuss the development of psychic skills and supernatural powers as a natural result of the spiritual exercises. Translations emphasised the development of the higher chakras echoing the desire to go beyond or escape from the bonds of the physical world. This false division into lower, mundane and higher, spiritual chakras misses the continually reiterated point in the original texts that all chakras are of equal practical value both in everyday life and in spiritual development.

Chakra imagery

Whatever their correlation to physical structures within the body, chakras are entirely non-physical. It is the mind rather than the sense organs that is the traditional tool for accessing and exploring the energy of each chakra. The main features of each chakra are described in the original texts in the same order as a meditator would mentally construct the necessary visualisation. Each image includes a god and goddess whose form and attributes encapsulate the inherent qualities that arise when the chakra is functioning in a balanced way.

The root chakra

Named *Muladhara*, meaning 'foundation', it has four vermillion petals around a yellow square. This represents the element of Earth and the four directions, north, south, east and west. Within the square is a downward pointing red triangle. The animal form representing the root chakra is a seven-trunked elephant. This shows solidity and assuredness. On the elephant's back rests the bija (seed) mantra – the sound that stimulates the energy of this chakra: *Lam* (pronounced with a short 'a' and a nasal 'nng' sound, rhyming with 'nun').

The sacral chakra

Called *Svadistana*, meaning 'sweetness', this chakra has six red petals around a crescent moon of light blue, representing the Water element. The animal is a crocodile – the sensuous, watery and deceptively strong energy of this chakra. On the crocodile rests the *bija* mantra: *Vam* (short 'a', nasal 'nng').

The solar plexus chakra

This chakra is called *Manipura*, meaning 'city of gems'. There are ten luminous blue petals surrounding a downward-pointing red triangle, the symbol for the element of Fire. The animal is a ram – headstrong and direct, his fiery nature controlling the group of which he is the leader. The deities represent control over anger and control of energy. The *bija* mantra is: *Ram*.

The heart chakra

The fourth chakra is *Anahata*, translated as 'unstruck'. It has 12 lotus petals of a deep red colour surrounding a hexagram – a six-pointed star of grey-green, representing the element of Air. The animal is a black antelope, leaping with joy. On the back of the antelope rests the *bija* sound: *Yam*, the sound here controls breath and life-energy.

The throat chakra

The fifth chakra is *Vishuddha* – 'pure'. It has a circle of 16 lavender or smoky purple petals enclosing a silver crescent and white circle of the full moon. This represents where all the elements dissolve into their refined essence, akasha – ether or space, the pure cosmic sound. The animal is an elephant, the colour of clouds. The elephant carries the *bija* mantra: *Ham*, which empowers the voice.

The brow chakra

The sixth chakra is *Ajña*, meaning 'command'. It has two petals of luminescent pearly blue. Within a white column, the 'colour of light' is a representation of unified consciousness – a combined male and female deity. There is no animal here – the *bija* mantra, *Aum*, rests on the finest quality of sound itself, known as *Nada*.

The crown chakra

Sahasrara, the 'thousand-petalled', is the seventh chakra at the crown of the head. Sometimes it is described as formless, sometimes as a moonlike sphere above which is an umbrella of a thousand petals with all the colours of the rainbow. The *bija* mantra is the 'nng' sound, known as *Visarga*.

Because they cannot be seen by normal means, the chakras and their related system of subtle channels are represented by diagrams and other symbolic maps of the body. This is necessary to clarify the relationship of the subtle centres to physical organs and structures with which we are familiar. However, this can lead to a very static, inflexible and two-dimensional view of what is an elegant, dynamic, ever-changing interaction of energies. Being non-physical, influencing matter but not consisting of matter, chakras are not bound by the laws of matter.

Physical correspondences

Near each chakra, echoing its function, is one of the main endocrine glands in the body, a concentration of nerves known as a plexus, and concentrations of blood vessels and lymph nodes. As the correspondences are not always linear, some discrepancy creeps into different systems of comparison, though there is general agreement of the relationships.

The root chakra

The first or root chakra is located at the base of the spine. In some systems the base is related to the testicles, in others to the adrenal glands. Although physically a long way from the root, the adrenal glands reflect the survival instinct of this chakra. The coccygeal plexus is the name given to the concentration of nerves in this area. This chakra is linked to the colour red in the rainbow system and yellow in the Vedic system.

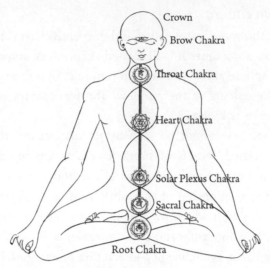

FIGURE 8.1 Positions of the chakras

The sacral chakra

The second or sacral chakra, sometimes called the sex chakra, is located in the lower abdomen, between the navel and the pubic bone. It is related to the sacral vertebrae in the spine, the sacral plexus of nerves and the sex glands – the ovaries and testicles. The chakra is associated with emotions and sensuality. This chakra is linked to the colour orange in the rainbow system and white in the Vedic system.

The solar plexus chakra

The third chakra is known as the solar plexus located on the front of the body between the bottom of the ribcage (diaphragm) and the navel. It is concerned with personal energy and power. The glands associated with this centre are the adrenals and the pancreas. The solar plexus chakra is named after the complex of nerves located here and is connected to the lumbar vertebrae of the spine. This chakra is linked to the colour yellow in the rainbow system and red in the Vedic system.

The heart chakra

The fourth chakra is the heart, located in the centre of the chest, associated with the thoracic vertebrae of the spine. The related gland is the thymus, a small gland above the heart, vital for growth and maintenance of the immune system. Two nerve centres that are located here are the pulmonary plexus and the cardiac plexus. This chakra deals with love and relationship. The heart chakra is linked to the colour green in both the rainbow and Vedic systems.

The throat chakra

The fifth chakra is the throat, located near the cervical vertebrae and the base of the throat. It manifests communications and creativity. The thyroid and parathyroid glands (controlling metabolic rate and mineral levels) and the pharyngeal plexus can be found here. This chakra is linked to the colour blue in both the rainbow and Vedic systems.

The brow chakra

The sixth chakra is the brow, in the centre of the forehead. This is linked to the pineal gland that maintains cycles of activity and rest, and the carotid plexus of nerves. The brow directs intuition, insight and imagination. This chakra is linked to the colour indigo in the rainbow system.

The crown chakra

The seventh chakra, the crown, is located just above the top of the head, though it influences all the higher brain functions. It is connected to the pituitary, the master controlling gland for the whole endocrine system. The entire cerebral cortex is influenced by this centre. The crown is associated with knowledge and understanding. This chakra is linked to the colour violet in the rainbow system.

Minor chakras, kundalini, nadis

The seven main chakras are only part of a much larger complex of subtle energies that make up the human being. There are many other chakras throughout the body and aura, all of which are expressions of different kinds of consciousness and energy. Surrounding each chakra are the main channels of energy or *nadis* that flow from the centre and interact with the rest of the body. These *nadis* do have a relationship with some aspects of the autonomic nervous system and also with the meridian channels but they are of a much finer subtle substance. There are said to be, in total, 72,000 *nadis*. Fourteen are named and described in detail, and of these three are of prime importance: the *ida*, the *pingala* and the *sushumna*. These three main channels run parallel to the physical axis of the spinal column. The *sushumna* is the central channel which is the most important.

Ida, the left channel, carries a lunar energy that is nourishing and purifying. *Pingala*, the solar channel on the right side of the *sushumna*, has a flow that is energising and strengthening. They are often shown in two ways; the first has all three channels running parallel to each other; the second shows the solar and lunar channels weaving between the chakras until all three meet at the brow chakra.

The fundamental life energy of the individual is thought to reside in a quiet state near the root chakra. It is called *kundalini*, meaning 'coiled up'. As the chakras and their *nadis* are cleansed of stress and other energy blockages, more of the *kundalini* energy can move through the body. As this energy is pure consciousness, its awakened state can create various degrees of realisation or enlightenment in the individual.

Many of the main chakras located on the central channel have smaller associated energy centres. For example, the *Muladhara* at the base of the spine has related centres at the groin points, the knees and the soles of the feet. All these help to ground and balance the physical energies. The heart chakra, *Anahata*, has a smaller chakra within it that has eight petals. This is the spiritual heart, the *Anandakanda*, whose eight channels represent the emotions.

The root chakra

The first chakra is located at the bottom of the spine and is the rock upon which the whole of the chakra system, the subtle energies and the physical body relies, and without which disorder soon arises. The Sanskrit name for this chakra is *Muladhara*, which means 'root'. Survival is the key activity of the root chakra, dealing with life at the level of practicality. It is our link to the planet itself.

This instinctive feel for survival is the 'fight or flight' response of the adrenal glands, the small organs that sit on top of the kidneys. The root chakra also relates to the skeletal muscles, the arms, legs and torso that allow us to move physically through the world and is responsible for maintaining the basic heat within the body – the core temperature that allows chemical reactions to take place in the cells at the correct rate.

The emotional responses of the root chakra are direct, explosive and strong, like anger, assertiveness and aggression, yet once they are satisfied, they dissipate immediately, Remaining in a constant state of alert drains the body's energy and actually makes it more difficult to respond effectively when real danger presents itself. Lust, physical passion and sexual excitement are complex emotions involving many different chakras. However, the motivation of survival of the species underlies the immediate physical attraction. A build-up of strong emotions, a tendency to selfishness, lack of any concern for others and a total withdrawal from emotions, all show imbalances in this chakra.

The root chakra is essential to manifest any idea, dream or concept. Without the down-to-earth energy it makes no difference how wonderful our inspiration is or how useful a new invention may one day prove to be. As soon as something takes its place in the real world, the job of the first chakra is done and unless supported by other energies, the creator will become quickly distracted by another new project. In a balanced root chakra there is energy, confidence, know-how and dexterity to survive and thrive in the moment-to-moment exploration of new territory. Root chakra imbalances at the mental level can show as obsessive focus, a rigid and materialistic outlook and deep insecurities about personal survival issues.

The spiritual purpose of the root chakra is the protection of individual integrity. The base holds together the fabric of the personality and is the very real foundation for every spiritual discipline.

The more someone works with spiritual growth and development, the more vital it becomes to anchor those energies. The root chakra is that lightning rod, that earth cable, which prevents the unwanted energies from destroying the individual's equilibrium.

GENERAL IMBALANCES IN THE ROOT CHAKRA

These include chronic lack of energy, exhaustion following even slight exercise, problems with the movement of the body, particularly hips, legs and feet, poor physical co-ordination, poor circulation (a tendency to have cold hands and feet), inability to relax the body, excessive tension or excitability, lack of drive or motivation, an aversion to getting involved in practicalities, a sense of confusion or unreality.

SPIRITUAL IMBALANCES IN THE ROOT CHAKRA

These include 'otherworldliness', a loss of awareness and interest in the real world and practical survival issues, a lack of discipline, an unfocused attitude, wishful thinking and fantasising, a disassociation from the body and its requirements, a desire not to be in physical incarnation, open to impressions, viewpoints and belief systems with little ability to discriminate, psychic impressions and clairvoyance with little or no control, a lack of grounding, hyperactivity, restlessness, inability to settle and very volatile emotions.

The sacral chakra

The sacral chakra is the second centre located in the area below the navel and above the pubic bone, the front of the pelvis. Physically, this chakra is involved with the organs of the lower abdomen – the large intestine, the bladder and the reproductive organs.

Detoxification is one of the key functions of the sacral chakra at every level from the physical through to the spiritual. Traditionally this chakra is connected to the element of water and it has those characteristics of flow, cleansing and movement. Any strain or tension here can create a whole range of symptoms from lower back pain, irregular or painful menstruation, constipation and sciatica to problems with fertility, impotence and fluid balance in the body.

Water absorption is a function of the large intestine, whilst control of the mineral/water balance in the blood is regulated by the kidneys. If the functions of these areas are impaired not only does the balance of chemicals in the body get upset, but it also becomes more difficult to get rid of toxins and waste products, effectively poisoning the body.

Once the needs of survival have been met the priority is to explore the potential of the body through play, and to explore the surroundings using all the senses. The sacral chakra maintains this flow of communication through feelings and emotions between body and mind. Vague intuitions and 'gut' feelings are often dismissed by the conscious mind because they are not precise enough. A balanced sacral chakra will accept more of these body-based assessments. Flowing in harmony requires flexibility and the ability to change focus – to let go, when necessary, of things that are no longer useful or helpful to us. Imbalance in this chakra often arises when, for one reason or another, we become fixated on something inappropriate or unrealistic.

Stress is any stimulus, good or bad, enjoyable or painful, that throws the body out of balance to such a degree that it is unable to fully return to its previous equilibrium. Stress initiates survival drives – first chakra functions. When stress is not able to be dissipated quickly by 'fight or flight' responses of the root chakra, the creative, flexible energy provided by the second chakra is needed.

Creativity is the natural state of life-energy and it restores life to natural balance. Successful art, beautiful design, skilful craftsmanship are exhilarating and life-supporting because they embody this flow of life-energy.

The sacral chakra is the focus of our experience of pleasure and it is the first place that experiences pain. Wherever trauma and pain may be in the body it is registered and held in the second chakra. Each event distorts or locks away energy that should be available for us to use in our everyday lives.

INDICATIONS THAT THE SACRAL CHAKRA IS OUT OF BALANCE

These include emotional over-sensitivity, unhealthy emotional dependency on someone else, a failure to respect normal boundaries with intrusive behaviour, rigidity with a lack of physical or emotional flexibility, repressed feelings, a fear of sensuality, sex, pleasure or enjoyment, guilt over one's feelings and desires, frustration and bitterness, upset of the physical functioning of the digestive system, particularly constipation, inability to become emotionally involved with life, a lack of enjoyment of life, being emotionally volatile, becoming aggressive or tearful at the slightest provocation, inability to let go of a stressful event so that it preys on the mind and suffering from an increasing number of infections and illnesses.

The solar plexus chakra

The solar plexus is conveniently considered as a single chakra, but, like most major chakras, it has many, close-related minor energy chakras. This concentration of energy is the third centre along the spine. Midway between the lower end of the ribcage and the navel, this centre also corresponds to the lumbar vertebrae in the spine. The physical attributes of the solar plexus chakra fall into three main areas: the digestive system, the nervous system and the immune system.

The process of digestion and assimilation of nutrients is vital to sustain life. The organs linked to the solar plexus are the stomach, liver, gallbladder, pancreas, plus the duodenum and small intestine. For digestion and the assimilation of food to be successful, all these organs have to work in harmony. The solar plexus is often referred to as the fusebox of the body. It contains large concentrations of nerve tissue that, if disrupted, can affect the nervous system throughout the body.

The immune system stores information about what the body has encountered. Problems with the identification of this information often show up when the body thinks that harmless, or even beneficial substances, are dangerous and instigates defensive reactions. Similarly, when the body harbours an infection for a long time because it fails to recognise its presence it fails to fight it at all. When the body fails to recognise its own enzymes, hormones or neurotransmitters, or when there is an inability to recognise minerals and vitamins that should be absorbed by the small intestine, these problems surface as deficiencies. However, the body will not respond to increased intake because lack is not the problem so much as a failure to recognise the substance.

The solar plexus chakra is put under great pressure by the way we live today. Its physical functions are strained by the types of food we eat, the pace of life and the new toxins in our environment. It is not surprising that many of the diseases in our society today are a sign of some dysfunction in the solar plexus chakra.

Issues concerning personal power are part of the solar plexus function. Fear can escalate into terror or subside into anxiety in any area of life. If people in authority use that dominant position to force us into habit patterns that take our personal power from us, the solar plexus chakra becomes effectively blocked. Failure to accede to this dominance is often met by criticism and punishment. Subsequently we may feel shame for this lack of compliance or skill.

Shame prevents us from working with this chakra at the emotional level, driving us into interacting with the world primarily through our thoughts. When the solar plexus chakra is functioning well, we are able to accept happiness in our lives. We can appreciate joy in the simplest of situations.

The solar plexus chakra working at the mental level is one of the most powerful tools we have at our disposal to create our circumstances, our own heaven or hell. It has been recognised by sages and philosophers for thousands of years that personal belief systems, the thoughts by which we recognise and understand how the world appears to work, are of critical importance.

Our body–mind catalogues and files away experiences and information for reference and retrieval as required and is able to identify things clearly and accurately, to label them correctly, to file them in the right place and to cross-index them where necessary. Confusion and fear often arise from false identification. Incorrect filing also creates confusion, learning problems and difficulties in retrieval (remembering).

If we are forced into certain learning situations before we are mature enough to cope, blocks around those issues occur and we develop negative belief systems about them. Beliefs will affect how we interact with the world around us and create disharmony in that relationship. Stresses build up and unless action is taken to correct the inaccurate beliefs, it usually results in physical, emotional and mental difficulties linked to the solar plexus chakra.

If we are unable to clearly identify events, our capacity to judge, weigh up alternatives and make decisions is very limited. Inability to learn or to study may be the result of forced or inappropriate learning situations in early life. Stresses once created here will be remembered by the body–mind every time a similar situation arises. If the stress around the events can be released, new learning strategies can emerge.

The solar plexus chakra at the spiritual level applies its energies to defining the boundaries of the self – the individual. The challenge at this level is to gain wisdom of the true nature of the self beyond the everyday level of persona. It is not possible to define who you are unless you can also identify who and what you are not. When you know who you really are, you can then begin to understand your place in the world. A major sign of progress along the path to wisdom is when there is an acceptance that the world does not owe you anything, that you are no more important than anything else in creation.

IMBALANCES IN THE SOLAR PLEXUS CHAKRA

These include inability to digest food, poor absorption of nutrients, difficulties with the stomach, liver, spleen, gallbladder, pancreas and small intestine; immune system difficulties, allergies and intolerances; restlessness and nervousness, fearfulness, worrying, confusion, poor memory, indecision, perfectionism and discontent.

The heart chakra

The heart chakra is located near the centre of the breastbone (the sternum). The physical organs and parts of the body linked to this chakra are characterised by their actions of expansion and contraction, drawing in and pushing away.

The heart, with its rhythmic expansion and contraction is the powerful muscular pump that sends oxygenated blood to all parts of the body. The diaphragm, the large muscle below the lungs creates, by its movement, changes in pressure which allows us to breathe in fresh air. As the diaphragm contracts, the outbreath expels carbon dioxide from the body. These processes of expansion, interchange and contraction are reflected in our relationship to the world. The relationship created is in constant motion; if stationary, all balance is lost.

The art of balance is a theme through all levels of the heart chakra. The element associated with this chakra is air. The experience of love is characterised by the flows of emotion, but for every falling in love there is a falling out of love. Trying to hold on to any fluid emotional state like love will lead to an obsessive, possessive attachment more reminiscent of an imbalanced sacral chakra response. Good relationships experience a constant falling in/falling out of love.

A balanced and coherent heart chakra is shown in the ability to accept ourselves, other people and all sorts of situations. Without a real self-acceptance there is no way that we are able to tolerate the foibles and faults of others. Relationships can be heaven or hell. In a balanced relationship, each person has autonomy, but both also share. In relationships that are unhealthy, love is conditional to the point of being a weapon to coerce the other into behaving or responding as required. Many of us experience this threatened withdrawal of love as small children, and until our heart chakras become truly balanced, we may continue to play out the same pattern on our own children, family and friends.

We inherit many of our thinking patterns in the same way. Dominant beliefs, especially negative ones, can be traced through successive generations. If we remain tied to these beliefs we never discover who we really are and independence is never really achieved. Rules may have been enforced in some way, to mould us into the person the maker of the rules had in mind. This process can create, for the most part, a fairly harmonious society in which to live but this type of thinking also has a robotic quality, producing members of the population who do not relate properly, where any interaction follows a set formula of etiquette.

Any repression and restriction suddenly becomes intolerable. Outright rebellion may seem to be the only way to break free of the suffocating pattern. The most desirable outcome is the development of a personal set of values and ethics that comes from a fresh, up-to-date perspective and that has a personal relevance.

At a certain point in the development and maturing of the heart chakra there is an opportunity to see oneself and the rest of the world from a very different perspective. The realisation dawns that while you can care, love and share with others you cannot live their lives for them or live your life through them. Everybody has their own personal path and unique direction in life. This releasing of another allows any possessiveness, misplaced sense of responsibility or dependence to disappear, allowing individuals to grow.

IMBALANCES IN THE HEART CHAKRA

These include heart and breathing problems, asthma, emotional dependence, depression, repression, inhibition, inability to relate to others, inability to share, agoraphobia, emotional manipulation, insecurity, lack of boundaries, lack of sense of direction.

The throat chakra

Language is the evolutionary leap that is often considered to be the major factor in the success of our species. Language has given us the ability to understand what is happening to others. The growth of society and civilisation is based on co-operation and a shared dream communicated by language.

The physical organs and structures of the throat area can be seen clearly as letting energy move through – either inwards or outwards. The mouth, nose and throat are where we first come into contact with the air around us. Even though the breath is initiated in the solar plexus we feel the air as it passes over the back of the palette and in the upper throat. The mouth and oesophagus come into contact with our food first of all – in fact vital digestive processes are carried out in the mouth. So much happens in this small area and it all has to be carefully regulated – we can only speak on the outbreath as air passes over out vocal cords; we must avoid breathing in at the same time as swallowing or we choke. Wrapped around the trachea and oesophagus are the thyroid and parathyroid glands. These major endocrine glands regulate the body's metabolism so that enough energy is produced from food for our needs. Lethargy and sluggishness result from an underactive thyroid and hyperactivity when it is overactive.

The voice allows us to express what is felt in the heart and mind. Blocks in our ability to communicate may not cause an immediate problem with the physical organs of the throat, but personal expression is deeply disturbing to the energy systems as a whole. It denies our existence, our individuality, our right to be heard.

Personal expression of ideas and thoughts, the ability to communicate through spoken language or the symbolic languages of writing, singing, performing or any of the other arts help to maintain the healthy flow of energy through the throat chakra.

As the body becomes more tranquil, mental activity also reduces and observant detachment becomes more apparent. With a balance of energies in the throat chakra, peace is a tangible experience, a familiar relaxed occurrence. Where the throat chakra is stressed or blocked in some way, peace may be a longed-for wish but it is difficult if not impossible to achieve. Expression and communication is this outward flow from the body via the activity of the throat chakra. If the expression is blocked in some way the energy will release through one of the other major chakras.

Communication is not simply about personal expression. It is also necessary to listen to what is being expressed by others. Problems also occur if individual expression has been stifled, often by overbearing discipline or unsympathetic schooling. To not be expressive simply because you believe that you 'can't paint', for example, is just reinforcing the same repressive values that have probably caused the problem in the first place.

Communication and sound are the keys to the throat chakra. Those who use these skills in their work are drawing on the energy of this centre. Communication by simple repetition has a tendency to break down very quickly, as the game known as Chinese whispers graphically illustrates.

The effective teacher is a person who feels excitement and interest and can express it to the students in a way that allows the knowledge to become their own, not simply repeated as inflexible dogma. Learning to explore alternative views, even taking up opposite viewpoints in debate, is a useful way of developing attitudes of flexibility and tolerance. Without these skills there is the danger that whatever is communicated to us will be automatically believed.

The throat is traditionally associated with the element of space, also called ether and, in the original Sanskrit texts, *akasha*. This fifth element was conceived as an original container, a vessel that held all the other elements. Creation myths often combine the moulding of inanimate matter with the life-giving addition of breath or with the process of naming. Naming myths and stories show the magical and spiritual significance of knowing the right names for things.

At its highest level the throat chakra brings out our own truth into the world. Truth is not just correct information. Each of us will dismiss as untrue those things that do not fall within our personal construction of how the universe works.

IMBALANCES IN THE THROAT CHAKRA

These include a stiff neck, throat infection or tension in the shoulders, headaches, problems with swallowing or eating, metabolic disorders, frustration that leads to shouting, or a complete withdrawal of communication, weak voice and rigid views.

The brow chakra

The chakra located in the centre of the forehead is *ajña*, meaning to perceive and to command. It is directly related to the senses of sight and hearing, although the upper three chakras – the throat, brow and crown – are all physically close together and share many correspondences. Throat chakra influences extend to the mouth, jaw and up to the ears whilst the brow has more links with the face, eyes, nose and forehead. The neck and base of the skull can be influenced by both the brow and throat chakras. Crown chakra energies relate to the cranium, the bones of the top of the head, approximately the hairline and above.

The consciousness of self, of unique personality of the mind is felt to be seated at the brow, like a commander at his control post. We are very much in our heads. The physical body belongs to us but it is not thought of as being us. With the awareness at the brow chakra, we begin to make sense of and interpret the world. The brow chakra is all about seeing, not just seeing with the eyes, but seeing with the mind – making sense and understanding what is being perceived. It is the brain that organises the visual information so that we can understand and really 'see' in a way that allows knowledge to become our own, not simply repeated as inflexible dogma.

Perception is the art of creating order from potential chaos, meaning from random impulses. Perception is the main function of the brow chakra.

Physical problems with the eyes can be helped by balancing this chakra. Clear seeing, understanding, perspective are all mental skills needed to interpret visual data as well as the mental pictures that are our thoughts, memories and ideas.

The brow chakra has a certain degree of detachment from emotional concerns. Silence and detachment allows the brow chakra to keep its perspective. Jumping to conclusions and making assumptions are signs that the brow chakra is becoming confused.

Detachment at the mental level gives the ability to step back from the normal waking experiences of time and space. The internal world of dreams, daydreams and the imagination are not limited to the rules of the physical universe. The brow chakra's language is light, a straightforward communication of energy that directly affects the electrical impulses of the brain, and from there, the whole system.

Intuition can be understood as a prompting from all the levels of awareness beyond the everyday conscious mind. Intuition presents a whole picture, an overview, an understanding that goes beyond simple explanation of parts. 'Clear seeing' or clairvoyance isn't necessarily only a visual experience, it is 'clear seeing' in the sense of clear, penetrating insight.

IMBALANCES IN THE BROW CHAKRA
These include headaches, eye problems, inability to relax, dislike of silence, constant daydreaming and lack of perception.

The crown chakra

The Sanskrit name for the crown chakra is *Sahasrara* – meaning 'thousandfold'. This refers to the image of the thousand-petalled lotus, given to that chakra that in Vedic thought represents the epitome of the human condition. The chakra is described as being just above the head.

The gland most often associated with the crown chakra is the pituitary, though some texts do quote the relevant gland as being the pineal. The pituitary gland is located at the base of the brain. It has two sections, the anterior and posterior, each responsible for releasing particular hormones.

The pituitary is often referred to as the 'master gland' because it affects so many body functions and other glands. The crown chakra, from the viewpoint of physical health, is mostly concerned with the co-ordination needed from the level of individual cells to ensure the smooth running of the bodily functions. The cerebellum helps us to co-ordinate our muscles for balance, posture and movement. The child who crawls on all fours helps to ensure that the nerve patterning in the brain is fully activated.

The development of expanded awareness characterises the crown chakra at the emotional level. The opportunity to begin to see and understand our individual role in the world does not present itself until our teenage years, as we begin to move away from a family base.

The drive to help others in the community and to be of service is a response to awareness of the needs of others. People expect this service to be truly selfless, but we often act because we may only feel useful if needed by others or we don't want to see the suffering of others. When there is a lack of awareness of our own personal requirements it is easy for the enthusiastic helper and healer to effectively martyr themselves to their ideals. Being emotionally attached to something is fundamentally an unwillingness to allow that thing to change, and such rigidity closes down possibilities. This can be faced and dealt with by being compassionate with oneself to let in all possibilities. Unless open compassion is primarily directed to oneself to allow healing at the crown chakra, it is impossible to be truly compassionate with anyone or anything else.

Thought processes associated with the crown chakra fall into two main categories: how we think the world operates and the thought processes linking us to the universal scheme of things. What we expect and what we fear has a knack of being drawn towards us in some way.

A natural maturing process initiates the search for greater knowledge. If this is seriously hampered by family, social and religious backgrounds that do not accept individual exploration, the crown chakra is prevented from working normally and it is unable to provide all the energy and information required by the other chakras.

A healthy crown chakra is a fine balance on all levels. Thoughts which come and go need to be treated in a way that appreciates that fact – they come and go. It is only when we hold onto thoughts without allowing alternatives or the possibility of change that disruption of the crown chakra happens. The more our consciousness expands the more we understand what we see, and so on, in a self-fulfilling, ever-increasing awareness.

The mind is a wonderfully restless, inventive and very slippery faculty to rein in, unless great understanding or cunning is used. Good meditation techniques offer a task for the mind to do to keep it occupied or engaged in a tight focus. The more we experience the gap between the thoughts, the more relaxed our bodies become and the more clearly we can see how our thoughts rule and shape our lives.

IMBALANCES IN THE CROWN CHAKRA
These include lack of co-ordination, constant self-martyrdom, delusion and inability to deal with the physical world.

Keeping the balance

The chakra system is a complex interrelated system where each chakra, both major and minor, can be thought of as a cog in a machine. A change in the movement of one will create changes throughout the whole structure. Locked together in their activity there will be an efficient flow of energy when all parts work harmoniously together. If one chakra, like a cog, becomes damaged or has its normal range of activity restricted this inevitably puts strain on its closest neighbours and its complementary chakra, which will also begin to suffer.

A chakra that becomes unbalanced has become stuck at an inappropriate level of activity. It is either working with insufficient energy for its task, or it is working too hard. In either circumstance the other chakras will have to compensate by changing their levels of energy. This means that the system as a whole will be working at one level when it may be more appropriate to function at another.

The chakra system, like the rest of the body, responds to the circumstances of its environment. Some activities will require a particular chakra to take a larger role, but this should still remain within the overall balance – within the normal working parameters of the system. Only if too much energy is focused in one area will problems start to show, beginning in those places where there are natural weaknesses from past stresses or strain in the present. Problems arise when, through stress of one sort or another the chakra system fails to change gear and becomes stuck in a single mode of functioning.

The more our energy systems are brought into harmonious balance, the easier it is to maintain that balance. Until some of the stresses can be removed from the chakra system every one of us will be so busy maintaining our false sense of equilibrium that there will be little spare energy with which to begin exploring our individual potentials.

As the ancient yogis of Indian and Tibet discovered, clearing the chakras from the build-up of age-old debris allows life to be entirely transformed – not into an escapist fantasy but the clarity of open, honest experience of the fullness of life where reality itself is completely satisfying and nourishing. In this state each chakra becomes a translucent doorway allowing a free flow of universal energies in and out of the body. False boundaries and the frustrating sense of separation dissolve because only the layers of stress and imbalance have created these distinctions in the first place.

The chakra system always works in two apparently opposite directions. From the root chakra upwards there is an increasing experience of expansion, from the focus and solidity of physical matter, through experience of sensation, personal power, expansion into relationship with the world, communication, understanding and finally integration on all levels at the crown chakra.

Simultaneously there is a flow of energy towards the grounding solidity of physical reality, from the timeless and directionless unity of the crown chakra to the defining vision of the brow, through the form-giving quality of naming, stabilising relationship between self and the world, learning how to control one's power, exploring the senses and finally being able to mould and create the raw material of the world – the practical energy of the root chakra.

In the same way that the individual chakras reflect and balance one another, each reflecting on the others in equal measure, so these two opposing tides are part of one unified process where expansion into the spiritual realms can only be effective with a reciprocal exploration into the universe of matter.

Working with essences, colour and the chakras

When listening to a client it may become apparent that their feelings, thoughts and description of sensations are highlighting issues linked to one or more chakras at one or more levels of function. The choice of appropriate essences can then come through use of the logical mind via descriptions of available essences or their colour correspondences and chakra links.

Having recognised the chakras that are related to what the client is saying, an assessment tool (pendulum or muscle testing) can then be used to determine which essence(s) are most appropriate for the client. A drop of an essence can be put onto a tissue or cotton pad to place onto the chakra.

The advantages of using chakras as an assessment tool are that they are multi-layered and it can be surprising easy to see how the client's words describe the functions and dysfunctions of a chakra. Colours link easily into chakras, making it easy to identify flower essences that might be useful.

The disadvantage of using chakras as an assessment tool is that the chakra system needs to be studied and well understood to make the best use of it.

EXAMPLE

Chakra clues that were picked up are in bracketed italics:

'James' came to visit for a therapy session, not specifically essences. He recounted his current situation as being one where he experienced very low levels of energy (*root chakra*). With careful prompting and questioning he admitted to having had an episode of what he thought was glandular fever several years before (*solar plexus chakra*). Initially he was very reluctant to talk about this as he had been told that what happened then had nothing to do with how he was now. The family saw it as his fault as he was prone to overworking (*solar plexus chakra and heart chakra*).

He said that he worried a lot about the future as he wondered how much longer he could continue providing for the family. He wanted to continue to do the best he could (*solar plexus chakra and crown chakra*).

Gentle questioning then led onto his daily routine. He said that he had noticed that after he had eaten his energy got even lower and he often wanted to go to sleep (*solar plexus chakra*). He had developed a tendency to work on the computer until late in the evening and then had difficultly falling asleep (*solar plexus and brow chakra*). This inevitably meant that he had difficulty getting up in the morning and it seemed to be getting worse.

Suggestions were these:

To stop working on the computer at 9pm and get to bed before 10.30pm.

To set the alarm clock for 7am and regardless of how he felt to get up and open the curtains and look out of the window for about five to ten minutes. This was to begin to reset the pineal gland and brow chakra and help the levels of melatonin and serotonin to become more balanced. This would take a while.

Essences suggested were (these were dowsed for):

yellow primrose (*root and solar plexus chakra*)

wild cherry (*root, sacral and heart chakras*)

yew (*root chakra*)

honeysuckle (*heart chakra*).

These were mixed to create a dosage bottle. Two drops, four times a day, to be placed on the palms of the hands, hands rubbed together and then cupped over the nose to be breathed in. This to be done for two weeks before coming for a second appointment.

Two weeks later James arrived looking a little better. He said that he had realised that he was addicted (*crown chakra*) to the computer! It was very hard to wean himself off. However, just the last two nights, he had slept better. He reported that his energy levels were more stable, although still very low. The wild fluctuations had gone (*root and solar plexus chakras*).

So began James' long haul back to wellness...

CHAPTER 9

SUBTLE BODIES
AND THE AURA

The chakra and meridian systems clearly define different functions and manifestations of energy in the body. Because of its simplicity and flexibility, working with the chakras has become one of the main techniques in healing. What is generally known as the human aura has been identified as a series of interrelated but discrete zones called the subtle bodies. There is less of a consensus on the exact structure and number of these energy bodies.

Most cultures describe the non-physical bodies in one way or another. Some have two or three, others have five or seven. It can be confusing to try to compare different systems, especially as the same names are sometimes used to refer to different things. All subtle systems, be they the chakra, subtle body, meridian or physical are to some extent models or maps and interpretations of how things really are.

Each system acts as a guide or map, but each is on a different scale. Using one energy map at a time reduces confusion. Mixing energy maps – using different systems simultaneously will often tend to confuse the outcome.

The subtle body system can be thought of as different aspects of the individual seen from particular perspectives and different vibrational rates. Each layer or level is as much 'us' as the physical self, but is not made up of solid matter. In much the same way as a normal photograph shows the external features of a person, whilst an ultrasound scan shows the internal organs and an X-ray photograph shows only the solid and bony tissues of the body, the subtle bodies represent finer, deeper and more subtle qualities of the self.

Described here is a model of seven subtle bodies, each level extending further from the physical body and constituted of finer energy material. It is important to remember that each succeeding level interpenetrates all the previous levels including the physical, so that there is a continuous, dynamic and complex interaction between them.

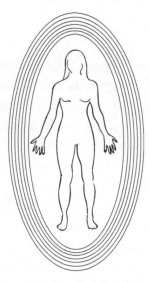

FIGURE 9.1 The subtle body system

The etheric body

The etheric body is the closest to the physical, and indeed it is considered to be the energetic blueprint upon which the cells and organs are built. It contains an exact energetic replica of the body with organs and structures the same. When imbalance and weakness occur in the etheric they will eventually manifest on the physical level, so in this respect the etheric body is the last line of defence against disease. Clairvoyant sight describes a blue or blue-grey web of ever-moving energy that extends a little way from the body. The meridian system is believed to be integrated with the etheric body or to act as the interface between the etheric and physical levels.

Offering healing energy to the etheric body will greatly accelerate the repair of physical tissues and may prevent other imbalances from gravitating into the physical body. The etheric levels are those that often tend to become misaligned from the physical body after shock and trauma. If this mismatch cannot correct itself, the physical body loses some of its organisational flexibility and this can allow disease states to take hold. Such etheric body dislocation may be the reason why in so many cases a serious period of illness follows a few months after significant shock. Any period of illness or recuperation would benefit from work on the etheric body. The etheric body has correlations to the colour orange.

The emotional body

The emotional body is the container of feelings. It roughly follows the body's outline but extends further than the etheric. It has no fixed structure and is composed of coloured clouds of energy in continual flux, altering with mood and emotional state. This field is often the coloured aura that sensitive people can perceive around a person. The emotional body holds our emotional and psychological stability and our sensitivity to those around us. This body is sometimes called the lower astral, or astral body. This should not be confused with the fourth level, here called the astral.

The emotional body is the closest vibratory level to the etheric and contains the volatile and ever-changing energy of our moods. It may be a useful comparison to see the emotional body as reflecting our own internal weather, continually changing in response to internal and external stimuli.

For such ephemeral feelings, emotions can play an enormous part in our health and well-being. Each nuance of mood affects the physical body chemistry and even the quality of life-energy that we are able to use.

Emotional balance is not an unfeeling, neutral state but a centre point to which the system can return between the extremes of happiness and sorrow. Without this fulcrum/balance/axis as a natural resting place, the emotions can get stuck in a mode of functioning that is inappropriate and deleterious to the body as a whole. Holding on to a particular sort of emotional energy disrupts the whole body weather system.

The mental body

The mental body is associated with thoughts and mental processes. It has greater structure than the emotional body and is usually perceived as bright yellow, expanding around the head during mental concentration. Thought patterns exist here as bright shapes coloured with emotion. It is in the mental body that we interpret information according to the belief structures that we have developed since birth.

It has quite distinct and discrete properties. The emotional body reacts, the mental body records, categorises and files these reactions. From birth it constructs how we understand the world and the way it seems to work. It uses all forms of information available to allow the individual to figure out what is going on. The mental body creates our core beliefs and then attaches all other experiences around these central 'truths'. Unfortunately, the core structures are created very early in life when the tendency is to believe everything we hear and often drastically misinterpret events and the actions of others. Because these structures are so fundamental to our self-image they can be difficult for us to see.

Core beliefs can exist in complete contradiction to each other so that when a certain issue arises in life, the opposite pictures of reality can create enormous stress in the body. This stress very often translates into muscular tension and physical rigidity. Easing mental body issues can allow relaxation at many different levels, from posture to tolerance of others' beliefs, to flexibility in problem-solving and finding positive options.

The astral body

The astral body is the fourth layer. Resembling the emotional body but with clouds of finer and more subtle colouring, this energy layer contains the essence of our personality. It is the boundary layer between the current individual personality and a more collective spiritual awareness, and is concerned with relationship, particularly between the individual and the collective.

It is the container that allows us to recognise ourselves as unique beings located in time and space. The astral body filters and tones down all other sources of energy and information so as not to swamp individual consciousness. It can act as a gateway both into physical manifestation and out towards expanded and collective levels of awareness. Weakness at this level can create great confusion in the perception of reality as the normal constraints of physical reality break down. Too closed an astral body, on the other hand, prevents useful information on other dimensions of energy from integrating into everyday consciousness, which can lead to feelings of unaccountable isolation and loss of direction.

The remaining subtle bodies

The three remaining subtle bodies are less often described and their functions are not so clearly defined. They certainly are composed of very fine energy.

The fifth layer is sometimes called the **causal body**, which links the personality to the collective unconscious and is the doorway to higher levels of consciousness. It patterns the experiences and lessons we have chosen to learn in life. The causal body can be seen, by analogy, as the projector that puts our own image onto the screen of physical existence.

The **soul or celestial body** is the sixth subtle level. It seems to focus fine levels of universal energy and is related to the idea of the 'Higher Self'.

The **spiritual body** is the seventh subtle body. It is the container and integrator of all other subtle energies. It has access to all universal energies, but maintains the individuality of each being. As the finest level that we know of, it is all-embracing, encompassing our whole existence in and outside of time and space.

Using essences with the subtle bodies and aura

Sweeping or spraying essences through the subtle bodies and aura can be very useful ways to change an individual's energy very quickly. Subtle debris trapped in the subtle bodies and aura can be removed quickly.

Once the essence(s) to be used have been determined, a few drops are placed in the palms of the hands. The palms are then rubbed together and then quickly swept through the energy field of the body (the aura) a few centimetres above the skin or clothes.

The advantages of these methods are that the essence is activated very quickly and very little essence needs to be used. This can also be done with specific hand and sweeping movements that can link to the meridian or chakra systems (see 'Meridian Massage' described in Chapter 10).

The disadvantages of these methods are that they are very obvious to an onlooker. Clients may not be familiar with the method and may be shy about using it or may doubt its efficacy.

TRADITIONAL CHINESE MEDICINE (TCM) AND THE FIVE ELEMENTS

About 5000 years ago, a complex system of examination, diagnosis and treatment was drawn together. Originally it was designed as a system of preventative medicine for the creation and maintaining of health, as opposed to dealing with things according to symptoms.

This system is seen as a healing art and science that looks at the whole human being – body, mind and spirit. It is a means of recognising the processes behind health and illness and therefore provides avenues down which to guide the restoration to health when illness occurs.

It sees illness as a collection of symptoms or signals that show distress. From a traditional viewpoint this would indicate a disturbance in the flow of prana or chi and so simply dealing with the symptom would be ignoring the real problem.

Several assessments can be done to uncover the problem, e.g. the colour of the face, the evident emotions, preferred tastes etc. Each organ in Traditional Chinese Medicine (TCM) is associated with a pulse and various facets of life that are seen as one coherent flow of energy. When this energy is disrupted it reveals itself in many ways.

Each of the Five Elements (Wood, Fire, Earth, Metal and Water) has a set of correspondences that help us to assess what is going on.

Everything in existence has an aspect of duality about it. We usually refer to these as opposites – dark–light, wet–dry, left–right etc. In fact, one cannot exist without the other, although one may be dominant at any given time. This is shown in the *Tai Ch'i Chuan* (commonly known as *YinYang*), representing a constant interplay of energies that moves in a cycle. Neither element of the duality is more important than the other. It is the same for the Five Elements.

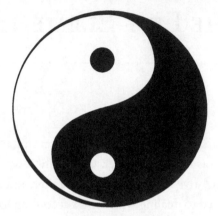

FIGURE 10.1 YinYang

Each element can be assigned a range of correspondences: colour, season, organs, time of day, direction, flavour, sense organ, emotion, bodily orifice, voice, odour, fluid secretion, food etc.

These help with the assessment of what is going on when health issues arise. In turn these indicate which meridians are out of balance.

This is only a brief overview of this huge subject; however it is enough to provide the practitioner with another energy model with which to work, alongside those of the chakras and subtle bodies.

TABLE 10.1 Relationships of elements with colours, seasons, directions, sounds, sense organs and emotions

Element	Colour	Season	Direction	Sound	Sense Organ	Emotion
Wood	Green	Spring	East	Shouting	Eyes	Anger
Fire	Red	Summer	South	Laughing	Tongue	Joy, happiness
Earth	Yellow	Late Summer	Centre	Singing	Mouth	Sympathy
Metal	White	Autumn	West	Weeping	Nose	Grief
Water	Blue	Winter	North	Groaning	Ears	Fear, phobia

TABLE 10.2 Relationships of elements with tastes, internal body parts, smells, climates, orifices and fluids

Element	Taste	Body parts	Smell	Climate that reflects the Element	Orifice	Fluid
Wood	Sour	Muscles and sinews	Rancid	Wind	Eyes	Tears
Fire	Bitter	Blood vessels	Scorched	Heat	Ears	Perspiration
Earth	Sweet	Physical body	Fragrant	Damp	Mouth	Saliva
Metal	Pungent, spicy	Skin and body hair	Rotten	Dry	Nose	Mucus
Water	Salty	Bones, bone marrow	Putrid	Cold	Anus, Genitals, Urethra	Saliva (teeth)

TABLE 10.3 Relationships of elements with external
body parts, body work, life aspects and foods

Element	External body part	Power, the capacity of the body to work with the Element	Life aspect	Foods that balance the Element
Wood	Nails, hands, feet	Control	Spiritual faculties	Wheat, peach, chicken, mallow
Fire	Complexion	Sadness	Spirit	Millet, plum, lamb, greens
Earth	Flesh	Belching	Ideas	Millet, apricot, beef, spring onions
Metal	Skin and body hair	Cough	Animal-self	Rice, chestnut, horse, onions
Water	Head hair	Trembling to create release	Willpower	Fish, peas, dates, pork, leeks

Table 10.4 shows important clues when listening to clients – timing
in the day/night when symptoms increase, occur or abate tell us
what elements and meridians are involved.

TABLE 10.4 Relationships of elements with meridians and timing

Element	Meridian (Yin)	Time of day	Meridian (Yang)	Time of day
Wood	Liver	1–3am	Gallbladder	11pm–1am
Fire	Heart	11am–1pm	Small intestine	1–3pm
Fire	Circulation/Sex	7–9pm	Triple warmer	9–11pm
Earth	Spleen	9–11am	Stomach	7–9am
Metal	Lung	3–5am	Large intestine	5–7am
Water	Kidney	5–7pm	Bladder	3–5pm

The meridian system

The meridian system of subtle energy is at the heart of TCM.
Knowledge of the meridians and the acupuncture points located

along them requires extensive in-depth study that can take many years. As such, most healers who are not acupuncturist or shiatsu practitioners rarely work with this system. There are, however, useful healing procedures that combine the energy of essences with meridian energies in quite straightforward ways. Once there is confidence in an assessment technique, such as dowsing or muscle testing, the correct choice of a specific essence on a meridian point can make dramatic changes to a person's well-being.

The meridian system, as devised by the Chinese, has 12 main energy channels that follow recognised pathways near the surface of the skin. Although it is one integrated system, each meridian has a starting point and an end point, which indicates direction of flow and function. Each meridian is named after an organ or function, such as liver or stomach, but this can be misleading as the physical organ is only a small aspect of the type of energy a meridian deals with. The functions ascribed to physical organs by the Chinese rarely have any recognisable Western correlations and it is important not to confuse these two very different models of the human body.

It has been generally thought that the meridians are non-physical, or etheric, vessels providing the physical body with the subtle nutrition of chi or life-energy. In 1962 research in Korea by Kim Bong-han suggested that meridians are, at least at some levels, superfine physical structures. This research was corroborated by Fujiwara and Yu in 1967 who were working in Japan. However, it was not until 2004 that this was confirmed by multiple studies in other parts of the world.

The acupuncture points along each meridian, often visualised as access points, or energy vortices, like small chakras, have been clearly identified as having a different electrical potential to non-acupuncture points. As well as the 12 meridians that flow on each side of the body, making 24 channels in all, there are many other vessels that feed the chi energy into smaller channels for distribution.

The most important extra channels are the conception vessel and governing vessel, both of which possess acupuncture points and flow up the midline of the body. These two channels help to maintain the flow of chi within the entire meridian system and directly affect vitality and health.

The meridians, their end points and emotional connotations

One simple way of understanding some of the functions of the meridians is to associate them with emotional states. Thus a positive emotion will energise or strengthen a meridian, whilst its corresponding negative emotional expression will tend to reduce the energy in the meridian. In this way it is possible to identify some of the underlying emotional energy causing disruption to the system. John Diamond, a pioneering kinesiologist, has discovered the attributions of the meridians and emotional states.

CENTRAL MERIDIAN (CONCEPTION VESSEL) [CV1–CV24]

Begins at the perineum and ends just below the lower lip.

Positive states are: love, faith, gratitude, trust, courage.

Negative states are: hate, envy, fear.

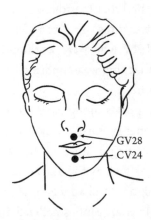

FIGURE 10.2 The central meridian and conception vessel

GOVERNING VESSEL [GV1–GV28]

Begins on the back at the base of the tail bone, rises up the spine over the head to the centre of the upper lip.

Emotional states are the same as for the central meridian.

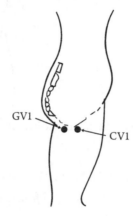

FIGURE 10.3 The governing vessel

LIVER MERIDIAN [LIV1–LIV14]

Starts at the outside of the big toe and ends at the bottom of the ribcage below the sternum.

Positive states are: happiness and cheerfulness.

Negative state is: unhappiness.

The liver meridian is paired with the gallbladder meridian.

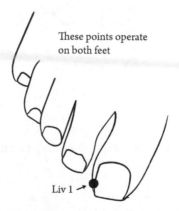

These points operate on both feet

Liv 1 →

FIGURE 10.4 The start of the liver meridian

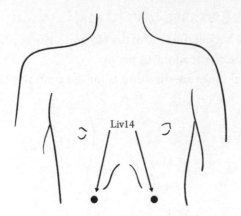

FIGURE 10.5 The end of the liver meridian

GALL BLADDER MERIDIAN [GB1–GB44]

Begins at the outer edge of the eye and finishes at the outer end of the fourth toe.

Positive states are: reaching out with love and forgiveness, and adoration.

Negative states are: rage, fury and wrath.

The gallbladder meridian is paired with the liver meridian.

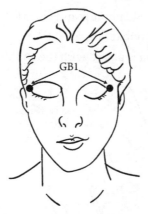

FIGURE 10.6 The start of the gallbladder meridian

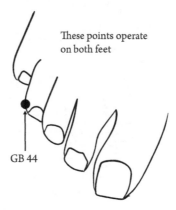

These points operate
on both feet

GB 44

FIGURE 10.7 The end of the gallbladder meridian

BLADDER MERIDIAN [B1–B67]

Begins at the inner canthus of the eye (against the bridge of the nose), and ends on the outer edge of the little toe.

Positive states are: peace and harmony.

Negative states are: restlessness, impatience and frustration.

The bladder meridian is paired with the kidney meridian.

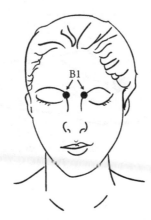

B1

FIGURE 10.8 The start of the bladder meridian

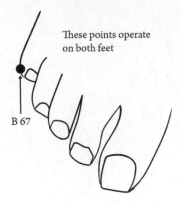

These points operate
on both feet

B 67

FIGURE 10.9 The end of the bladder meridian

KIDNEY MERIDIAN [K1–K27]

Begins at the ball of the foot and ends where the collar and breastbones meet.

Positive state is: sexual assuredness.

Negative state is: sexual indecision.

The kidney meridian is paired with the bladder meridian.

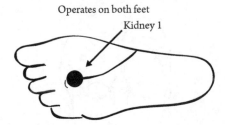

Operates on both feet
Kidney 1

FIGURE 10.10 The start of the kidney meridian

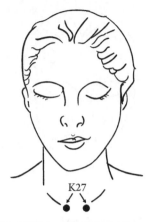

FIGURE 10.11 The end of the kidney meridian

LARGE INTESTINE (COLON) MERIDIAN [LI1–LI20]

Begins on the inner end of the index fingers and ends on the face by the outer edge of the nostrils.

Positive states are: self-worth, acceptance.

Negative state is: guilt.

The large intestine meridian is paired with the lung meridian.

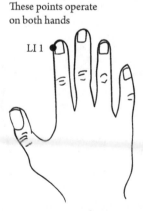

FIGURE 10.12 The start of the large intestine

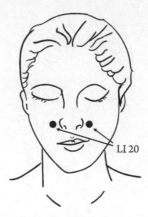

FIGURE 10.13 The end of the large intestine meridian

LUNG MERIDIAN [LU1–LU11]

Begins just below the corocoid process on the shoulder and ends on the inner end of the thumb.

Positive states are: humility, tolerance and modesty.

Negative states are: disdain, contempt and prejudice.

The lung meridian is paired with the large intestine meridian.

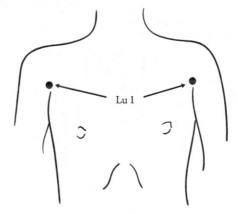

FIGURE 10.14 The start of the lung meridian

These points operate
on both hands

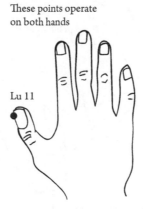

Lu 11

FIGURE 10.15 The end of the lung meridian

STOMACH MERIDIAN [ST1–ST45]

Begins below the eye at the inner edge of the orbit, and finishes at the outer end of the second toe.

Positive states are: contentment and tranquillity.

Negative states are: disappointment, disgust, bitterness, greed, nausea, hunger, emptiness.

The stomach meridian is paired with the spleen meridian.

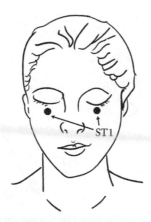

FIGURE 10.16 The start of the stomach meridian

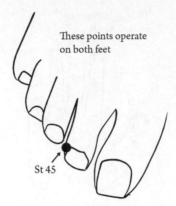

These points operate
on both feet

St 45

FIGURE 10.17 The end of the stomach meridian

SPLEEN MERIDIAN [SP1–SP21]

Begins at the inner edge of the big toe and ends at the side of the ribcage just below nipple level.

Positive states are: faith and confidence about the future and security.

Negative states are: realistic anxieties about the future.

The spleen meridian is paired with the stomach meridian.

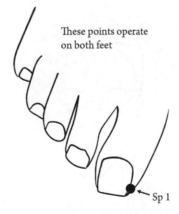

These points operate
on both feet

Sp 1

FIGURE 10.18 The start of the spleen meridian

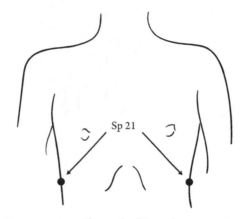

FIGURE 10.19 The end of the spleen meridian

CIRCULATION–SEX MERIDIAN (PERICARDIUM, HEART PROTECTOR) [CX1–CX9]

Begins at the outer edge of the nipple and finishes at the inside end of the middle finger.

Positive states are: relaxation, generosity, renouncing the past, letting go.

Negative states are: regret, remorse, jealousy, sexual tension, stubbornness.

The heart protector meridian is paired with the triple heater meridian.

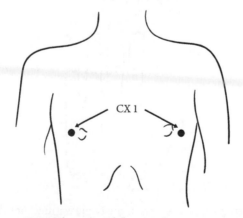

FIGURE 10.20 The start of the circulation–sex meridian

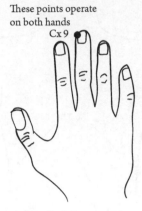

These points operate
on both hands
Cx 9

FIGURE 10.21 The end of the circulation–sex meridian

TRIPLE WARMER MERIDIAN (TRIPLE HEATER) [TW1–TW23]

Begins at the outside end of the ring finger (third) and ends at the outer edge of the eyebrow.

Positive states are: elation, hope, lightness, buoyancy.

Negative states are: loneliness, despondency, grief, hopelessness, despair and depression.

The triple heater meridian is paired with the heart protector meridian.

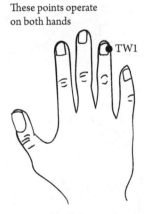

These points operate
on both hands
TW1

FIGURE 10.22 The start of the triple warmer meridian

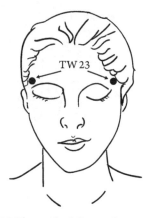

Figure 10.23 The end of the triple warmer merdian

HEART MERIDIAN [H1–H9]

Begins at the forward edge of the armpit and ends on the inner edge of the little finger.

Positive states are: love and forgiveness.

Negative state is: anger.

The heart meridian is paired with the small intestine meridian.

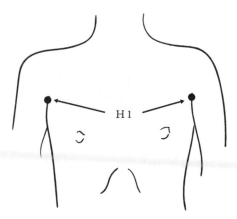

Figure 10.24 The start of the heart meridian

These points operate
on both hands

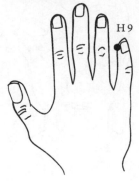

H 9

FIGURE 10.25 The end of the heart meridian

SMALL INTESTINE MERIDIAN [SI1–SI19]

Begins at the outer end of the little fingertip and ends at the upper edge of the ear in a small hollow of the cheek.

Positive state is: joy.

Negative states are: sadness and sorrow.

The small intestine meridian is paired with the heart meridian.

These points operate
on both hands

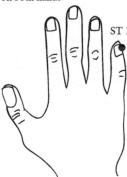

ST 1

FIGURE 10.26 The start of the small intestine meridian

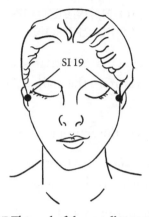

FIGURE 10.27 The end of the small intestine meridian

Working with essences and the meridian system

Meridian massage

Meridian massage is a quick means to bring an overall balance back to the body. It can be used with another person and for oneself. It quickly restores energy levels and can reduce a range of symptoms, emotional, mental and physical.

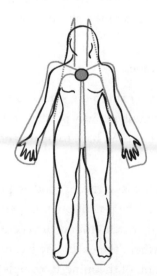

FIGURE 10.28 Meridian massage

PROCEDURE FOR DOING MERIDIAN MASSAGE ON ANOTHER PERSON

1. Ask the person to stand comfortably with legs slightly apart and arms held away from the body, palms down and towards the body.

2. Place a few drops of the appropriate essence(s) on the hands.

3. Begin with both hands over their heart area. Keep an inch or two away from the body throughout.

4. Sweep up to their armpits and along the insides of the arms to the hands.

5. Pass over the fingers and return up the outsides of the arms to the shoulders, meeting again at the throat.

6. Sweep both hands up the face and over the head, following as closely as possible down the midline of the back and then down the outside of the legs to the feet.

7. Pass around the toes and up the inside of the legs and then on up the midline of the torso to the heart. This is one circuit. The number of circuits and the speed of movement is a personal choice.

8. Repeat several times.

9. Ask the person to turn to the side so that the process can be completed by simultaneously passing both hands up the front and back midlines from base to upper and lower lips, at least three times.

When doing meridian massage on another person, they will be standing to the front of the practitioner. Depending on size it may not be possible to fully reach around the client's back. This is not too important – anywhere the exact line has to be departed from, simply use the intention of the mind to complete the sweep across the appropriate area.

HOW TO MERIDIAN MASSAGE ONESELF

1. Start with the right arm extended, palm up, and the left palm on the centre of the upper chest.

2. Sweep the left hand down the inside of the right arm, around the finger tips and up the outside of the right arm to the back of the right shoulder and return to the upper chest.

3. Repeat steps 1 and 2 with the left arm extended and sweeping with the right hand.

4. With both palms placed on the upper chest, sweep both hands upwards over the nose and top of the head and down to the back of the neck.

5. Place both hands, behind the back at kidney level and bring the hands down over the hips, down the outside edge of the legs to the front of the toes.

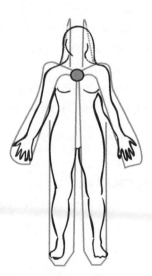

Figure 10.29 Self meridian massage

6. Pass the hands in front of the toes and up the inner legs, sweeping up the torso to the upper chest. This is one circuit.

The number of circuits and the speed of movement is a personal choice.

7. Complete the process by simultaneously passing one hand from the pubic bone up to touch the lower lip and the other hand moving up the spine from the coccyx as far as it goes. Then move that hand to reach down the spine (as if retrieving an unseen thread) and then pass over the back of the neck, top of the head and down to touch the top lip.

8. Repeat several times.

The advantage of this method is if there is a general need to strengthen the meridian system, it is better to use techniques such as 'meridian massage'. A balanced meridian system usually means that, taken overall, there is not a lack of energy or an excess of energy in the system. Individual meridians, or parts of meridians, may be working outside of their normal ranges, but in a balanced system a general equilibrium is kept by any excess in one area being balanced by a lack in another. Like every other subtle system, and even the physical systems of the body, a small change in one area may create a larger effect overall. It is not possible to isolate a part from the whole.

The disadvantage of using meridian massage is that it can look strange to the client at first; however, when its efficacy is recognised, this is released.

Colours of the elements

The colours of the five elements can be matched to the colour correspondences of the essences, especially to flower essences.

Direct use of colour

When listening to the client it may become apparent from the description of their problems or from the times of the day that the issues seem to worsen, that one or more of the TCM elements is being activated.

Using logical assessment, intuition, dowsing or muscle testing, the appropriate essence(s) can be determined for the client.

The advantages of this method are that it is straightforward and easy to implement as long as the colours of the flower, item, crystal or environment are known.

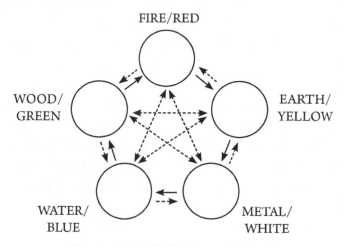

FIRE/RED

WOOD/
GREEN

EARTH/
YELLOW

WATER/
BLUE

METAL/
WHITE

FIGURE 10.30 The direct use of colour

The disadvantages of this method are that it may be unfamiliar to the client and they might doubt its efficacy.

Sequence of colour

Use of essences could also be used to mirror the *sheng,* the creative cycle of elements, clockwise, or the *ke (ko),* the destructive, controlling cycle, or cross-centre relationships. There is also the unwinding cycle of elements (anticlockwise). The latter, the 'unwinding' cycle is not used in TCM, but is used in energy work to 'unpick' anything that has been created that is causing dis-ease states.

In the *ke* or destructive and controlling cycle when problems arise within an element that overpower the element, it may be appropriate to use an essence linked to the colour of the controlling element to ease the situation.

The *sheng* cycle is the process that manifests into the physical world. Using a series of five essences using sequential processing (one drop of each essence in sequence) in the colour order of the *sheng* cycle and determining which colour starts the cycle can be useful in creating new beginnings.

The 'unwinding' cycle is the process that unpicks what has been created. This is useful for complex situations that have become entrenched and where the whole being needs to restart or de-programme an issue. Here a series of five essences using sequential processing (one drop of each essence in sequence) in the colour order of the unwinding cycle is used having determined which colour starts the cycle off.

The advantages of these methods are that they are fast in creating energy change in the client and they are very useful for clients who are very familiar with essences or other alternative and complementary techniques.

The disadvantages are that the client may be unfamiliar with the technique and may doubt its efficacy.

Specific meridians

This is a procedure for working with essences on a particular meridian. The 'end points' as these points are known, are where the meridians reach the surface of the skin. Working with these points creates a general balancing effect along the entire meridian being focused upon:

1. Having determined that it is appropriate and safe to work with a meridian, find out which meridian is involved, either by dowsing or muscle testing.

Remember that, apart from the central and governing vessel, all meridians are in pairs, that is, there is one on the left and one on the right. Only one side may need to be worked on.

2. Determine which side of the meridian pair needs balancing or if both sides require attention.

3. Determine which of the end points of the meridians you have found in step 2 need essences.

4. Check to see if essences are needed at one end only or both ends of the meridian, and if the latter, whether different essences are needed.

5. Find which specific essences will rebalance the meridian(s) indicated.

If dowsing, the use of categories or lists can be very useful. If muscle testing, broad categories and lists can be useful.

6. Determine how long the essence needs to be on the point(s).

7. Introduce a drop of essence to that point(s), either directly onto the skin, onto a cotton pad, tissue or onto clothing at that point.

8. Once the process is completed, recheck that everything is in balance as sometimes other meridians will show they need work when one has been adjusted.

9. Make sure the client is fully grounded and suggest they drink a little more water than usual for a few days to help the adjustment process.

The advantage of this method is its speed in creating energy change in the client. The disadvantages are that the client may be unfamiliar with the technique and may doubt its efficacy.

SPECIFIC MERIDIAN POINTS

If meridian maps are available, it is possible to deliver an essence to a specific meridian point. Knowledge of the meridians is needed to do this in a logical manner, but dowsing and muscle testing can be used to determine what is appropriate, following a similar pattern to working with a specific meridian (above).

This is a very powerful method to deliver essence(s) to a client and is excellent for removing stubborn blocks on any level. The disadvantages are that good meridian maps are needed and they are not easy to obtain. The client may also be unfamiliar with the technique and may doubt its efficacy.

USAGE

A drop of an essence can be put onto a tissue or cotton pad to place onto the meridian point.

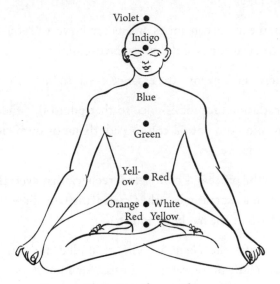

FIGURE 10.31 Specific meridian points

CHAPTER 11

COLOUR CORRESPONDENCES

Each colour signifies an energy frequency of light with very specific properties and effects. Everything is affected by colour. Plants, animals, bacteria, food and chemical reactions are all affected by colour. Change the colour that something is exposed to and the behaviour changes.

Colour is a universal, subconscious language. So it makes no difference whether we know what a colour signifies or what effect we think it will have. Every colour automatically creates physical, emotional, mental and chemical responses in us. The colours of a flower, crystal, landscape or any other item an essence might be created from give the primary clues to the effect that essence is likely to have on the majority of people.

A secondary level of colour is the learned or conditioned response that comes from the particular culture and society we live in.

Linking the seven main chakras with the seven colours of the visible or rainbow spectrum is therefore not an old system, but it works very well and it is easy to remember. Early in the 20th century the fascination with the significance of the number 7 (as in seven visible planets, seven days of the week, seven main chakras or energy centres in the body and seven colours in the visible spectrum), became a major theme in alternative spirituality, largely based on Theosophical ideas.

The original Vedic system of colour correspondences of the chakras works in a slightly different way, referring to elemental colours. The main differences are that the root chakra in the Vedic system is yellow, the sacral chakra is white and the solar plexus chakra is red.

Cross-linking colour with chakra and five-element information builds an energy dictionary and structure of information exchange that can be useful in dealing with the issues that clients bring into a session.

Red

Red throughout history has had a connotation with life and those things generally considered sacred in some way. Red ochre found at ancient burial sites hints at the hope for a renewal of life. The colour red has become synonymous with the preservation of our life-force, as in the logos of the Red Cross and Red Crescent. Danger signs and signals are also often surrounded in red or coloured red to indicate warning of the loss of life.

Red is the colour with the longest wavelength of visible light. It is the nearest visible light to infra-red in the electromagnetic spectrum. Although red occurs beyond the infra-red, it still has close connections with heat and warmth. Even rocks will become red when they are heated sufficiently. This is seen in volcanic eruptions when lava pours out onto the surface of the earth.

Fire, too, has these two facets. It can be a warming life-saver or an uncontrollable destroyer. In our daily lives, too much red energy will harm or exhaust us, too little and we have no energy for any activity. Too much red energy and we become over-involved in the workings of the material world and with too little we could find the world a threatening and dangerous place that we would feel the need to escape from.

Physical level

Red at a physical level relates to the circulation of the blood through the body that provides our cells with oxygen (fuel) and nutrients (food). To maintain red energy we need to exercise and eat in a way that maximises this to the full. If we eat too little or continuously exhaust ourselves physically and mentally, not only does this process falter, we also place too much stress on our adrenal glands. These glands control our ability to respond to survival situations by pumping hormones into our bloodstream, heightening senses and reaction times. If we abuse our bodies for too long, this natural reaction becomes a permanent state, which eventually leads the whole system into a state of collapse. Typical 'red' exercise involves using the lower limbs – walking, running, swimming or bicycling, which, when carried out for about 20 minutes, increases the oxygen supply to our cells. Massaging the legs or feet can do the same. Eating red coloured foods and foods rich in minerals can increase the amount of energy that is available to us. The effect of red on the eye is quite unusual. For the colour to be seen, the eye itself makes internal adjustments. This alteration means that we see red objects as closer than they really are.

Emotional level

Any direct expression of emotion is linked to the colour red. Anger and passion, especially, have both traditionally been thought of as 'red' emotions, and phrases like 'red rag to a bull' and 'red in the face' have crept into everyday speech to reinforce this. The characteristics of 'red' emotions are their strength, their immediacy and their short duration. Black and red are the colours most associated with evil entities, for example the archetypal 'red devil' of medieval artists. Blatant expression of emotion is not always easy to handle, whether it is sexuality, passion, anger or aggression. When expressing red emotions, the heart beats faster, the capillaries dilate and the skin becomes flushed and feels warm.

Many societies avoid or refuse to accept the expression of these emotions. This produces people who feel guilty about being angry or deny their passion. Wearing red clothing or carrying red crystals can help to overcome this or it can sometimes be easier to introduce something red into the living space. Flower essences such as scarlet pimpernel, hazel or oak can also be used to ease the expression of red feelings.

Mental level

On a mental level, the drive to start new projects and to create foundations for new business is related to red. The energy that creates innovators and entrepreneurs is seldom adapted to the management of stable businesses, so the initiator will often leave once the new project is working. It is not uncommon to see combined with this level of initiative a very assertive character who needs to be impulsive, rash and daring. They must continually challenge or test themselves to reinforce their living and survival skills. Often they are also renowned for daring exploits and can be somewhat extrovert and boastful about their skills.

Red is 'immediate'. This immediacy affects the thinking processes causing restlessness and impatience. It can result in selfishness, focusing on personal needs and survival above everything else. Sometimes this drive to survive is what fuels impulsive actions and rash comments.

When mental energy is low, visualising red or eating red energy foods can help (e.g., coffee and tea are both 'red' energy), though too much increases irritability and can create addictive behaviour.

Spiritual level

On a fine, spiritual level, red reminds us that no matter how spiritually inclined we may be, we are dependent on the survival and well-being of our physical body to act as a tool to express that spirituality in the world. Wearing red, eating red foods or foods rich in minerals, exercising, releasing our strong feelings and occasionally acting on impulse all reaffirm our connection through our bodies to the material world.

Life should be grabbed and lived with a sense of immediacy. Without red we become listless and out of touch with reality and we fail to live our dreams in this world. Without the foundation that red gives us we can daydream of escaping into non-existent realities and events. Without the support of our planet, also a red energy, we as a species will neither succeed nor survive.

Summary: To increase or balance the red energy in life

Wear red clothes.

Eat red coloured foods or foods that supply red energy (remember – coffee, tea, sugar and chocolate are only temporary red 'fixes').

Use red crystals: garnet, red jasper, ruby.

Use essential oils that have red energy: ylang ylang, frankincense, black pepper.

Use flower essences of red flowers: scarlet pimpernel, red rose, hazel.

Activities: running, speed and field sports.

Chakras: Linked to the root chakra and the solar plexus chakra.

Element: Linked to fire.

Orange

Orange is created from a blend of red and yellow in equal parts. The yellow content gives the powerful red energy a capacity to be directed and sustained. Orange has two qualities that carry through its functions on all levels of our being. These are release and creativity, linked by the need for life-force to flow through us completely unhindered. Like fire, orange energy displays some sense of direction and purpose – it moves along the pathways that fuel its own existence. Orange is certainly dynamic, but more thoughtful and controlled than explosive red.

Physical level

In the physical body orange is related to the lower abdomen in general, but to the large intestine and reproductive organs in particular. The large intestine deals with the ability to release by the elimination of waste products. The reproductive organs are concerned with fertility.

Without the ability to release waste products from the body efficiently, the system becomes constipated and toxic. Eating orange foods (apricots, oranges, carrots) and foods that relate to orange qualities (brown rice, foods high in natural roughage, oats), can reduce the incidence of such problems. Massaging the lower abdomen and back with oils that carry an orange vibration (neroli, sandalwood) can help to relieve symptoms. The ability to create something real from our dreams, ideas and inspiration works through the orange energy. The bodily function of reproduction is only one facet of this creativity. Children of the emotions, the mind and our dreams are also gestated and born here. Musicians, artists and dancers all use a lot of orange energy. When creative energy gets blocked it can be released by using orange. Wearing orange, eating orange foods, massaging with 'orange' oils and orange items within the environment will all ease the flow of energy. Flower essences from orange-coloured or orange-smelling flowers, such as marigold and mock orange can also play their part. When a system becomes static or blocked, not only is constipation present on all levels, but there is lack of creativity too. If the physical symptoms in either area persist, the underlying emotional and mental problems linked to orange need to be addressed.

Emotional level

Orange on the emotional level links the extremes of fun and pleasure with shock and trauma. When we shut off the enjoyment of life for any reason, orange in any form can be a difficult colour to settle with. Strict social mores concerning personal pleasure, desire and enjoyment, repress and inhibit the flow of orange energy through the body, creating blocks of guilt on all levels – physical, emotional, mental and spiritual. The same effect occurs after experiencing trauma, particularly if we felt powerless. In these cases, orange can be uncomfortable as it tends to remind us that something needs to be dealt with. If orange can be introduced carefully, in any form, it can bring about the healing that is needed. When we are unwilling or unable to let go of memories or problems, we can experience a sort of emotional constipation and excessively tense muscles. This can lead to the physical problem of constipation, urinary difficulties and tenderness in the lower abdomen or back.

Whilst red is a focusing or self-centred energy, orange reaches out to see what it feels like to be somewhere else – it is the toddler reaching for everything and wanting to taste everything. Orange is learning to experience the world with a sense of play, enjoyment and exploration.

Mental level

On the level of the mind orange releases the creativity of the universal artist. This is not just about formulating ideas, but bringing them to fruition in a way that enhances beauty and elicits appreciation from others. This can be achieved through any medium so long as it brings pleasure, release and relaxation. Orange represents instinctive (rather than intellectual or thought-out) problem solving. This sort of orange energy is manifesting when someone is working on the design of their garden. It can also emerge through a potter working clay, or an artist sketching a design, or a poet scribbling down ideas. Even doodling on a pad whilst listening to someone on the telephone is exhibiting the natural urge to explore through creativity – allowing a flow of energy to balance the sense of identity.

Spiritual level

On an even finer, spiritual level, orange represents the subtle blueprint of our physical bodies, often referred to as the etheric layer, or that part of the aura that is closest to the physical body. In this layer, the model for our physical body is held. If our physical, emotional or mental bodies become damaged, the etheric does too. Effective healing will repair the etheric. If the etheric is not repaired, pain can remain or the physical body never completely heals because the template (or model) is incomplete. Use of any sort of orange will keep the energy and information held in the etheric free of blocks, leaving the physical body to complete its healing and to release stress effectively.

A balance of orange energy brings a willingness to get involved, to 'get one's hands dirty' with practical exploration. It allows us the ability to fill time creatively and to be aware of the needs of the body.

Summary: To increase or balance the orange energy in life

Wear some orange clothing.

Eat orange foods (oranges, apricots, peaches) or foods that create an orange effect (brown rice, oats, sesame seeds, Vitamin C, zinc).

Use orange crystals: carnelian, dark citrine or crystals that work in an orange way (dark opal, Herkimer diamond, selenite).

Use orange essential oils (neroli, mandarin, cedar).

Use flower essences made from orange flowers (marigold, Californian poppy).

Activities: music, dancing, any form of art.

Chakra: Linked to the sacral chakra.

Gold

When a mix of red and yellow favours the colour yellow, the rich tones of gold emerge. Our instinctive reactions to gold shows us, possibly more than any other colour, how universal human responses to colour are. The mineral gold has been sought after or fought over (on the battle field and in the boardroom) because acquiring vast amounts is indicative of wealth and status. Gold is a commodity that powerful people would like to control as its rarity reflects those qualities of 'work' and 'value' that are most highly regarded.

Physical level

The colour gold when shone onto the body soothes nerves and encourages the body to relax, as does the visual impact of the colour. Minute amounts of the mineral gold are required for optimum functioning of the nervous system. Gold resonates to the skin, the largest organ of the body, and creams made from gold-coloured flowers (chamomile, marigold, evening primrose), and gold-coloured natural oils (vitamin E) are used to heal minor damage to the skin and to help to keep the skin supple.

Emotional level

The links that gold has with our emotions highlight the qualities of contentment and comfort. Wearing gold brings a degree of self-awareness and confidence that gets people noticed. In small amounts gold can suggest wealth and good taste, whereas too much hints at a vulgar need to impress. This demarcation between a class act and a shyster showman is very subtle. Individuals through the ages have all fallen foul of what is acceptable and what is judged as pride and boastfulness. In a state of balance, gold can create and project a lazy emotional style that is a comfortable and secure place to be.

Mental level

There is a natural leadership quality associated with gold at a mental level – to be a successful leader there has to be an ability to carry the weight of the inevitable attention, preferably without the ego becoming too large. If the balance of gold is lost, an egotistical, proud dictator emerges who, ironically, denies everyone else of their own gold qualities of happiness, relaxation and contentment. It is important not to get complacent with success but to somehow keep it fresh and untarnished. Taking time out to play and have fun is an important part of gold energy – rekindling joys of childhood and the appreciation of natural beauty.

Spiritual level

At a spiritual level, outsiders looking in see a serene, wise and well-rounded personality. It is easy for the onlooker to assume that since gold energy at a spiritual level 'has it made', there is nothing else to be achieved. What they fail to realise is that like a swan on a pond, the elegant vision of ease hides furious paddling. Gold at this level shows that a constant vigilance and hard work directed to self-development and self-healing has got results, but it also never stops.

Summary: To increase or balance the gold energy in life

Have something of golden colour in your immediate environment.

Eat foods that bring warmth to the body – spicy foods, ginger.

Take time out to play in the sunshine.

Wear gold jewellery, amber, rich citrine, gold topaz.

Use herbs and nutrients like Vitamin E, dandelion.

Chakra: Linked to the solar plexus chakra and the crown chakra.

Element: Linked to earth.

Yellow

The bright, crisp yellows have an invigorating effect compared to the cosy shades of gold. Yellow is linked to the ability to make decisions from the given information. This is not just a mental function, it works through all aspects of our lives. The richest source of yellow is the light from the bright sun (in the main part of the day). If we exclude natural light from our lives, for whatever reason, we cut ourselves off from one of the greatest sources of healing.

Most people will recognise the sensation of warmth and vitality when looking at a strong pure yellow. Like the energy of a bright sunny morning yellow brings clarity to our awareness. As with all colours, the type of yellow will create markedly different responses. An orange-yellow or golden colour imparts a sense of establishment, of solidity and assuredness, a rich, round sensation of inner warmth. A clean, clear yellow seems to clear the mind whilst keeping it alert and active in a state of readiness. An acid yellow is stimulating and enlivening, whilst a shade of yellow with just a touch more green will create discomfort, disorientation and even nausea.

Physical level

In our physical bodies yellow relates to our digestive, nervous and immune systems. All of these systems depend on the correct information being available and the subsequent correct choices being made. Our digestive system breaks down the food we eat into constituents that our bodies identify and absorb for our health and growth. If the digestive system's decisions go awry we experience digestive problems and poor absorption of nutrients. The nervous system relays information to our brain where it is sifted, filed and acted upon when necessary. If the nervous system cannot prioritise, confusion and fear increase. The immune system identifies and destroys cells it considers harmful to the body. If the immune system mis-identifies cells, we can find ourselves failing to fight viruses, bacteria and other invading cells or identifying harmless items as something that needs to be fought (as occurs with allergies) or, at the another extreme, fighting our own healthy body cells by mistake (auto-immune diseases). Many of us need extra yellow to combat the pressures of living in the 21st century. Wearing yellow may not always popular, but yellow in our homes, yellow foods, food supplements and herbs that resonate with yellow (Vitamin B, evening primrose oil, Vitamin E, St John's Wort) can all help.

Emotional level

Emotional issues can easily upset the physical embodiments of yellow. Fear and anxiety, both for known and unknown reasons, can have debilitating physical effects. Conversely many people who find themselves mentally and emotionally stressed can be so as a result of problems created by imbalances in physical body areas sensitive to yellow issues. Unfortunately we live in an age where information dominates our society and the processes of logic and science are considered vital. We work in artificial light often surrounded by electrical machines. All of this depletes yellow energy. As the body becomes more stressed, thinking processes start to fail. Without yellow it is difficult to concentrate, study or remember things we are aware that we know. Enhancing yellow helps the ability to discriminate and judge what is needed. Without a balance of yellow at an emotional and mental level, we strive for an unreachable perfection instead of accepting our best efforts.

Mental level

The functions of the yellow vibration have to do with decision-making, with what to do in any given situation. Decisions rely on information but more importantly on the ability to decide which bits of information are relevant.

The nervous system relays information to the brain that then categorises, interprets and acts upon the signals. Correct identification of priorities leads to an easy relationship with the world. When this yellow function is lacking, confusion and indecision creeps in. Fear and worry are the consequence of an imbalance of yellow energy, born of wrong information and a lack of clear and logical thought causing an inability to act positively.

Society in the West is currently very focused on the yellow qualities of acquisition of knowledge, organisation, structure and information exchange. The senses are continually bombarded with information from the environment, advertising, music and the media as well as new foods, new chemical substances and different energy sources. Many people, too, work in completely artificial lighting conditions behind tinted glass under fluorescent light. As a result many people need additional yellow light to help them keep the balance in their busy lives.

Spiritual level

Spiritually, yellow represents the ability to know who and what we are. With this ability we can deflect the unwanted attention of others and unwanted energy from machines in our environment. If we cannot differentiate between ourselves and our surroundings, we become entrained in a world dominated by things outside of ourselves, and we feel powerless and weak.

Summary: To increase or balance the yellow energy in life

Wear yellow.

Introduce yellow into your surroundings.

Eat yellow foods (bananas, grains, citrus fruits), and foods rich in vitamins.

Supplement the diet with Vitamin B complex, Vitamin E, St John's Wort or evening primrose oil.

Sunbathe for short periods.

Use crystals: lemon quartz, yellow citrine, yellow fluorite.

Use flower essences from yellow flowers: daffodil, crocus, marigold, chrysanthemum, hypericum.

Chakra: Linked to the root chakra and the solar plexus chakra.

Element: Linked to earth.

Green

Our eyes are especially sensitive to all shade and tints of green. Green is in the middle of the visible spectrum and epitomises the qualities of balance and harmony. It is the colour we relate to Nature, trees and plants and to a way of life that works in harmony with the Earth.

In Nature, we see the physical expression of green in the new shoots of plant growth in the spring. This is part of the natural cycle of birth and death that we readily accept in nature but can have problems accepting in ourselves. The processes of life and growth inevitably involve the death of one cycle, so that another can emerge. This creates the balance. For any growth and development to be sustainable, each stage builds on what has gone before. When we have problems working with or accepting this, a walk in a park, a forest or by the sea can bring back our perspective. Whether vegetarian, vegan or carnivore, we all depend in some way on the plant kingdom for our food. Reverence for all life helps to keep our perspective in harmony with reality.

Physical level

In our physical bodies, green relates to the heart, lungs, the arms and hands. The heart and lungs are organs that rhythmically expand and contract, in a cycle of renewal and elimination that we depend on to live. The arms and hands we use to pull things and people towards us, for closer inspection, to hold or relate to. We also use them to push things away from us when we feel we no longer want or need them in our lives.

Emotional level

Emotionally, green is expressed through the way of relating to everyone and everything in the environment. This is a balance of personal requirements with the needs of others. In personal relationships this dynamic is an ever-changing set of polarities. We seem to explore these extremes before settling on the balance – weighing freedom against inhibition and repression, caring and love against manipulation, control and dominance against encouragement. Learning how to relate to others is a skill of balancing our needs with the needs of the other person. If it is possible to develop a mutually agreeable relationship of caring and sharing, both lives are enriched and expanded – our interaction with the world is broadened. When a relationship is formed that is negative, manipulative or unpleasant in some way – very often because one person is trying to gain power and control over the other (a negative green tendency) – then our own potential for understanding the world is curtailed and restricted.

Emotions constantly change and we can be misled if we expect emotions to be the same all the time. Like the heart and lungs, the process of letting go and holding in never stops. Security cannot be achieved emotionally, as emotions fluctuate as part of their natural function.

Mental level

Mentally, green teaches us the patterns and cycles of our thinking processes. When we are young, we take our guidance and behaviour models from those who set the rules. This is fine as it helps us to become secure in our homes and immediate surroundings. As we mature, we reach a point where we need to take on the process of setting our boundaries and patterns of behaviour ourselves, accepting the new responsibility that comes along with it. Breaking away from the patterns and ties of childhood is not easy, but unless this happens we are unable to grow into independent adults. It is usually better for this 'breaking away' to happen when there is a chance to take a break from the normal flow of our lives, as this gives time to explore the new possibilities. At these times wearing green can be very supportive. Many people instinctively bring more green into their lives at these times – even eating only green foods for a few days can encourage changes in our thinking.

Spiritual level

On a spiritual level, green reflects the capacity to 'do your own thing' regardless of what everyone else says or does. Far from being deliberately eccentric or rebellious, this confirms that at this level we are unique. No-one can live our lives for us. We can take advice, but ultimately we are responsible for ourselves. Accepting this can free an individual, which in turn gives the opportunity for others to release themselves from any duty of care they might feel they had for that person. Everyone can then move on to the next phase of growth. The green energy inevitably has to do with the pushing out of boundaries, of growing beyond what is known. Because it is expansive it must develop relationships with those things around it, but it is also necessary to also have some degree of control and power.

This power can be expressed in a harmonious way, as in an ecological balance where all elements are accommodated and mutually supportive, or it can be destructive to everything around it, simply absorbing or taking over, enforcing new order upon others.

Summary: To increase or balance the green energy in life

Wear green clothes.

Eat green foods (leafy vegetables, apples, pears etc.).

Walk in the countryside, around trees or sit in the garden.

Use crystals: e.g. aventurine, emerald, green jasper, jade, tourmaline.

Use flower essences made from tree flowers: e.g. lime, maple, willow.

Use any essential oils.

Chakra: Linked to the heart chakra.

Element: Linked to air and wood.

Blue

Blue is the colour of distance. When artists of the early Renaissance began to consider how to represent perspective, they employed the simple observation that in nature the further away an object was in space, the more 'blue' it appeared. Naturally, blue in this way is associated with looking beyond what is in the immediate environment – stretching the perceptions outwards beyond the known.

Gazing at a sky on a sunny day or at the stars on a clear night, the blues – one bright and one very dark – can both instil wonder, peace and an appreciation of the vastness of space and the universe. Across all bands of experience, blue indicates a flow of energy. There are two aspects of blue. On the one hand there is the experience of going beyond what is known – searching for information or detail, the process of communication, and on the other hand the experience of rest and peacefulness – simply happy to be experiencing without any particular focus of thought. In some respects these seem to be contradictory qualities but in fact the uniting factor is the desire for equilibrium.

Physical level

Blue has a sedating effect on the physical body. Shining blue light onto the body has been used to reduce inflammation and swelling in joints and other tissues. It will calm any situation down when used for short periods. If used in lighting for too long, though, it can become depressive and cold. Blue is also linked closely to communication of all sorts. The most common sort is verbal communication – language, speech, singing and laughter – but it also includes non-verbal skills and body language. When communication of any sort is prevented or inhibited the natural flow stops. This creates a build-up of pressure, which we often experience as frustration or disappointment.

Since blue is related to the ears, eyes, nose and throat, inhibiting the flow of energy can create physical problems in these areas. If you are prevented from speaking out, sore throats, ear-ache and a stiff neck could be the physical result. If this should occur, wearing a blue scarf or tie around the neck or carrying blue crystals can reduce some of the more uncomfortable symptoms. Arnica, the classical homoeopathy remedy for trauma, acts as a 'blue energy', as it brings flow into a situation that has become stuck through shock.

Emotional level

For thousands of years blue has been associated with objects or people of devotion (the Virgin Mary and Krishna). Here devotion is directed towards a powerful emotional source. This flow of devotion can bring the attributes of these beings closer to the lives of people. Blue can also calm our emotions, allowing thoughts to separate from ordinary levels of communication. Many old places of worship have blue stained-glass windows or blue décor to help this process along.

The colour blue somehow seems to free the thought processes from their normal activity, removing us slightly from involvement with thought, emotion or physical activity. A 'cool' personality avoids getting caught up in emotional turmoil or any particular belief. That distance is the same quality as the blue of the distant mountains –

not overwhelmed by detail or closeness, having the possibility of greater perspectives.

Mental level

The flow of mental energy and communication related to blue moves to provide a clarity of knowledge and understanding. Both teaching and learning, especially associated with philosophy, religion and further education, are linked to blue. Blue therefore becomes an ideal colour to wear if you want to instil confidence in others and to be thought of as someone who is reliable and trustworthy.

All kinds of communication like talking, listening, hearing, learning and the exchange of information and viewpoints are blue activities. So too, are the expressive arts – not just the performers such as actors, singers and musicians, but any art form that seeks to make itself known to other people. All is communication of information, and any of the five senses can be used to tell the story or carry the message.

Spiritual level

Sometimes the speed of information is such that we can have sudden ideas or intuitions that if followed, will change our lives. These seem to come from outside of our normal mental functions, and are sometimes thought of as coming from the Infinite or Divine. Blue represents the realms of subtle perceptions at a fine level. These skills include clairvoyance (clear seeing), clairaudience (clear hearing) and clairsentience (clear feeling). Skills such as mediumship and the ability to channel information from other sources also relate to the darker shades of blue. All of these can be seen purely as an information flow from one source to another, but from a more unworldly source than day-to-day communication and conversation. For these types of skills to become secure and stable, the energies of the complementary colour orange and the grounding energy of red are both needed.

Summary: To balance or increase the blue energy in life

Take time to look up a clear blue sky on a sunny day.

Wear blue clothes.

Introduce small amounts of blue into your environment.

Use essential oils like rosemary, lavender, blue chamomile.

Use flower essences from blue flowers, e.g. bluebell, harebell, forget-me-not, scabious.

Use crystals, e.g. celestite, blue topaz, sapphire, blue lace agate.

Chakra: Linked to the throat chakra.

Element: Linked to water and space.

Indigo

There is a different quality to the experience of looking at a midnight blue or indigo sky. Indigo amplifies the characteristics of blue in a profound, resonant way. At a physical level, for example, whilst blue is quietening and cooling, indigo is sedating. In a depressed state indigo is to be avoided as it can easily deepen the depression.

In a way, indigo turns the energy of blue inwards: while blue creates flow between people by some form of communication, indigo creates an internal communication that manifests as profound thought processes, new insights, philosophy and intuition. The flow of blue can be fast, but the flow of indigo can be almost instantaneous, often leading to the sensation of ideas 'coming out of the blue', with no previous development or build-up of thoughts and ideas. Intuition and sudden clarity of awareness, startling realisations and innovative concepts occur in this 'super-cooled' state of indigo.

Indigo is related to all the subtle perceptions such as clairvoyance, clairsentience and clairaudience (clear seeing, feeling and hearing) as well as other psychic skills. The deep, directionless depths of indigo can sedate the conscious mind enough so that more subtle, delicate perceptions can be noticed. Blue energy is the skill of language and eloquence – the narrator. Indigo energy, on the other hand is definitely the listener. Blue energy can be frivolous and superficial, indigo energy will be profound and significant.

The internal quality of indigo and the enhanced sense of removal from normal, everyday communication can mean that those using a lot of indigo energy are able to step away from how the world is usually seen and come up with new, startling ways of thinking. The inventor has these qualities, going beyond the consensus view of what is possible and often appearing to be socially out of step or isolated. The internalising qualities of indigo make it an ideal colour to use in contemplative and spiritual contexts, particularly where the emphasis is on solitary meditations and attention to internal communication such as the practice of visualisation where the inner senses become more important than the physical sense mechanisms. Without the qualities provided by indigo we would need to find other resources to help provide deep quietude in our lives.

Summary: To balance or increase the indigo energy in life

Take time to look up at a starry night sky or take time to be alone and silent.

Wear dark blue clothes.

Introduce small amounts of dark blue into your environment.

Use crystals, e.g. sapphire, lapis lazuli, sodalite, azurite.

Chakra: Linked to the brow chakra.

Element: Linked to water (double-water).

Violet

Hundreds of years ago, violet and purple dyes were very expensive commodities and were reserved for use by the ruling classes, the clergy and the rich. Today shades and tints of violet are often thought of as the 'most spiritual' colours, mostly based on their historical use. For well-being, though, we need all colours and no one colour is more important or spiritual than any other. The tradition that links violet with healing is explained by its blend of red and blue, the opposite ends of the visible spectrum. A body will take from violet light the energy it needs, so violet can be applied in any situation to help to create well-being.

The key to understanding the energy of violet is to see how its component colours work together. Red is a focusing, concentrating, dynamic and activating energy, whilst blue is a cooling, quietening and expansive energy. Violet brings a new dynamism to the unfocused expansion of blue and a stabilising energy to the frenetic activity of red. The rather undirected spaciousness of blue is made practical by the addition of the red. Concepts and ideas are thus better able to find some real application in the world. The energy brought by red allows more creative qualities to emerge from the blue, thus violet is associated with the imagination and with inspiration.

Physical level

Violet is related to the head. Its constituent colours of red and blue can represent the different and opposite functions of the left and right hemispheres of the brain. The left hemisphere is linked to logical thought and outward expression, the right hemisphere to creativity and absorption of information. The degree of balance between the hemispheres is seen in the individual's ability to co-ordinate physical movement and other activities that need the left and right sides of our body to work in synchronistic harmony.

Emotional level

The emotions that resonate with violet are seen in those who work with selfless service for others. Sympathy and empathy and the ability to see other people's points of view are very noticeable. Violet, however, also seems to also show the opposite facet of its energy very easily. This is apparent where people martyr themselves for others, not with a healthy and altruistic stance, but from a lack of value in themselves. Helpers can see others as more needy or deserving and so sacrifice themselves. Viewed from a broad perspective, this is a type of negative-egotism.

A more balanced standpoint is to help others to the maximum of one's ability as well as looking after your own well-being. Then the help and service can be carried on indefinitely as it is coming from a stable emotional base. The complementary colour to violet, yellow, and its quality of self-knowledge, helps to stop the violet energy from becoming unwieldy.

Mental level

The ability for violet to highlight the extremes of its vibration is most apparent in how it manifests at a mental level. As a beneficial quality, violet is the colour of imagination and inspiration. Sometimes, all too easily, these positive traits can sour and become fantasy and delusion. Holding the positive balance requires input from all the other colours of the spectrum and their accompanying skills. The sleight of hand of the magician can amaze, yet that same skill in a trickster can disgust.

Spiritual level

Violet as a spiritual energy projects the integration of the spiritual aspects of life into the mundane and practical. Many teachers and gurus tell us that it is pointless having high ideals and views if we cannot apply them in our daily lives. This is the challenge of violet. Bringing these two together is easiest through some sort of ritual. Whatever you choose to do – regular attendance at a place of worship, daily personal prayers or giving thanks for a beautiful day – when done from the heart with sincerity, is very powerful. Incense, special clothes and specific foods can all create a sacred space to connect and integrate with your inner being. Violet is an important energy to those who use the blue and indigo skills of psychic perception because it helps to supply the grounding energy for the work. Without the anchoring abilities of red, the use of subtle perceptions can seriously imbalance and exhaust the life-energy of the practitioner.

The skill of integration is aided by violet. As the colour combines opposite energies, so it can help people who also need to work with an array of disparate things. Violet is often associated with the richness and diversity of ceremony, perhaps originating from its ability to psychologically balance the minds and actions of the participants.

Summary: To increase or balance the violet energy in life

Wear violet clothes.

Use crystals: amethyst, sugilite, violet fluorite, diamond, charoite.

Use essential oils: lavender, violet.

Use flower essences of violet flowers: violet, pansy, petunia, lavender, gentian etc.

Examine your motives for getting involved in healing, charities and groups.

Chakra: Linked to the crown chakra.

White and black

When people speak of opposites it is usually in terms of black and white. Strictly speaking neither are colours – simply characteristics of the presence or absence of light. In a way, both white and black reflect the attitudes of the individual. In a person with a lot of fear and uncertainty, black is a threatening unknown, a silence in which one's own terrors and nightmares can be amplified. In another person, black may simply be experienced as a restful emptiness that allows many different possibilities to emerge and disappear back again.

As in all polarities, black and white cannot be defined without each other. Like day and night, white and black are part of an unceasing definition of existence.

White

White is what we humans perceive as the entire visible light spectrum seen together – the complete energy of light. In this sense it stands for wholeness and completion – nothing has been taken out, everything is present. In many cultures white is associated with purity and cleanliness, openness and truth. When everything is shown in bright light, nothing is hidden.

This also relates to the way white can be used to denote holiness. White is also the colour of bone and the snow of winter so for some, the energy of white relates to the starkness of death and endings. Both of these interpretations, purity and death, are connected by the act of setting things apart from normal life, creating a sense of specialness. Entering or leaving the world, white signifies beginnings and the end of one cycle enabling another to start.

White is uncompromising. Everything is clear, open and explicitly manifest. It has a cold quality. White can be of use when clarity is needed in life. However, it can take on the hue of other colours around it and so acts a little like a mirror to the energies in proximity. White can be a rather uncomfortable colour for those who do not wish to have their hidden feelings reflected back to them.

As a vibration of purification, white can help to clarify all aspects of life, giving encouragement to sweep away blocks in physical, emotional and mental patterns. In the same way that there are no shades of white, the action of this energy can be uncompromising and rapid.

Wearing white can be a deliberate device to set oneself apart from or above others, making any approach difficult and therefore possibly creating unnecessary fear or suspicion. The addition of a small amount of another colour to white will make a huge difference to the response from others.

The core energy of white is direct and impersonal. It can represent rapid transformation and complete change as it sweeps away blocks on all levels of being. Its ability to purify what it contacts is unsurpassed. Without another colour to soften it, white can be an uncomfortable experience. Flower essences made from white flowers (star of Bethlehem, stitchwort, daisy, snowdrop) can help to create profound changes in emotional and mental patterns. Clear and white crystals tend to work in the same way and are excellent transmuters and transmitters of energy.

Summary: To increase or balance the white energy in life

Wear white with another colour of your choice.

Fast for a day, drinking only water.

Use clear and white crystals: e.g. clear quartz, moonstone, opal, diamond.

Use flower essences of white flowers: star of Bethlehem, cherry laurel, daisy, snowdrop, apple, nettle.

Chakra: Linked to the sacral chakra.

Element: Linked to metal.

Black

White reflects all aspects of light, black absorbs all aspects of light. So whilst white reveals, black conceals. In the simplicity of symbolism white is translated as whole, holy and good, so black inevitably becomes linked to the hidden, fearful and bad experiences. Black is the fear of a starless, moonless night – everything is unseen and unknown – anything might be hiding out there to wish us harm. Where white is seen as the colour of emergence, of birth and change, black is then the colour of continuity, of withdrawal from any definition, of the hidden. White continually makes its presence felt: it shouts 'I am here!' Black withdraws into the background, refusing to take a stand or be noticed. Black has often been associated with the energies of the Earth and the fertile soil. Black represents the rich earth from which all life and sustenance springs as well as the same earth into which the dead are placed.

Instinctive reactions to black suggest an innate response to this absence. For some, black is to be feared, representing emptiness, evil and a void that touches a hidden place deep inside. To others it is a safe, impersonal haven where individuality can be safely lost.

Physically, black creates a holding energy that, depending on the situation, can be a help or a hindrance. It absorbs all forms of energy. Wearing black clothes keeps someone safe from the unwanted attention of others. This creation of a protected shield allows the wearer to go unnoticed in their immediate surroundings. As soon as a splash of colour or decoration is added to black, the anonymity ceases and the black serves to highlight and enhance the individual and their appearance.

Emotionally, black can provide a respite from many strong emotions. By reminding us of the impersonal darkness of night time and the safety of womb-like places, black can create an energy into which to withdraw. For short periods this can be very healing. Deeply held emotions that have been buried can be brought to the surface to be dealt with. All through our lives, when we fail to fully experience the pain within a situation, the unprocessed emotions get locked into our 'Shadow Self'. This is sometimes called our 'dark side' because we know it holds the sum of all our painful emotional baggage.

Mentally, black shows the hidden depths of our mind. This can also be related to the Shadow Self, to the thoughts that unconsciously direct our lives. When thoughts are allowed to arise and fade without attention paid to them or action taken on them, the mind reflects the pure potential of black. Many people do not allow themselves enough quiet time to experience this aspect of the mind. When attention is first turned within there can seem to be a barrage of thoughts that some may perceive as outside of themselves or as a result of some maleficent influence. Filling time with activity and constant stimulation effectively cuts off the awesome depth and potential of the mind, and denies us access to that part of our Shadow Self. In this way we do not get the chance to discover our hidden skills, whilst many unacknowledged thoughts and fears are projected onto others for them to act out, so we can blame others for our own shortcomings. Taking time out by ourselves, to become familiar with our own company and our thoughts can ease all this. Sitting quietly with eyes half-closed, allowing thoughts to come and go, paying no attention or giving no encouragement, helps to experience black at a mental level.

Spiritually, black is the exploration of the depths of the mind. By allowing the mental quality of black to become an everyday experience, the emptiness of the mind holds no fears. When thoughts do arise, their beauty and the clarity of the perception of those thoughts carries a spark of joy in creativity that is unsurpassed.

Summary: To balance the black energy in life

Spend time alone, practising 'being' rather than 'doing' or thinking about 'doing'.

Use black crystals: smoky quartz, obsidian, black tourmaline.

Chakra: Linked to the brow chakra and the Earth Star (a chakra point equidistant below the feet as the root chakra is above the feet).

Element: Linked to water (double-water).

Turquoise

Turquoise is a blend of green and blue. It is so named because the Turks were fond of the colour and decorated many of their buildings in turquoise ceramic glazed tiles. Turquoise has the calming, expansive nature of green and the cool, quiet flow of blue. It can remind one of the skies just before sunrise and after the sunset, the sea, a mountain stream or a distant natural scene.

Physical level

Turquoise creates an easy flow of energy through the physical body that helps relaxation, not just physically, but also emotionally. Working particularly on the upper chest, turquoise can help to deepen breathing and relax tense muscles in and around the shoulders and upper back.

This in turn, helps the thymus gland to function correctly, aiding our immune system to withstand the onslaught of the pressures of living in the present day. Restriction of natural behaviour patterns and the inability to find one's place in the community causes a rapid build-up of stress and toxins in the body. This leads to a decrease in energy and greater susceptibility to disease. Turquoise can help when there is low energy, lack of interest in life, a failure to fit in with the surroundings or a lack of courage to strike out on your own.

Emotional level

On an emotional level, turquoise helps the true expression of personal emotions. The energy of turquoise allows the expression of our wishes. The green quality of growth is added to the blue quality of communication. This is not a 'lip service' type of expression, but one that reflects the true individuality of each person. For many, this aspect of turquoise is difficult to accomplish. Wearing turquoise coloured clothes or bringing the colour into the home as furnishings or wall colour can help if self-expression is a difficult thing. The resurgence and popularity of this colour in the 1990s reflected the growth in diverse spiritual philosophies.

Mental level

Mentally, turquoise epitomises the opportunity to express or interpret old ideas in new and relevant ways. It can be a useful colour when one needs to take a stand over an important issue or when it seems difficult to fit easily into one's surroundings.

Spiritual level

On a finer level, turquoise is very protective. The mineral turquoise has been greatly valued in the parts of the world where it occurs naturally. Historically it has been used both as a protector and healer. Wearing a turquoise amulet or piece of jewellery can also help heal issues associated with all aspects of the colour.

Summary: To increase or balance turquoise in life

Wear some turquoise coloured clothes.

Wear turquoise jewellery or carry a piece in your pocket.

Try to say what you feel and not what you think people want to hear.

Chakra: linked to the small chakra just above the heart chakra (near the thymus gland).

Pink

Pink is red and white combined in varying degrees. The quality of its energy will depend on how much of the energy-supplying red vibration is present. White is the potential for fullness, red is the motivation to achieve that potential, therefore pink is a colour that promotes personal energy in the context of the whole.

Pink is sometimes seen only as a soft, feminine colour, a colour representing the qualities of caring and tenderness. It will certainly help to take the heat out of any turbulent or aggressive situation. The dynamic mix of red and white is a useful balance of male/female energies that can also be useful as a healing colour, reducing the effects of disease as well as the fear and anguish disease can cause. Whereas violet balances the spectrum extremes of red and blue, pink harmonises the gender polarities of male and female, or *Yang* and *Yin*, expressive and receptive.

Emotional and mental levels

Pink helps to support an underlying confidence to existence. Such a level of support means that pink has the ability to neutralise negative or destructive tendencies. Aggressive behaviour patterns arise where there is fear at an emotional level or irritation and friction at a physical or mental level. Pink provides sufficient energy to move out of that negative state and enough clarity to understand and clear away misconceptions. The paler pinks link more closely to attitudes we hold about ourselves, e.g. self-worth, self-tolerance and self-esteem. Many people are able to express love for others more easily than they can for themselves. Forgiving others often comes more easily if we have come to forgive ourselves first. A high level of self-acceptance comes from facing the fears we have about ourselves.

Deep shades of pink that veer towards magenta have proved to be extremely effective in situations of disorder and violence, such as in prisons and police cells where a limited exposure to pink light rapidly removes aggressive behaviour. These deeper shades of pink can help to improve self-confidence and assertiveness, while the paler shades are more protective, peace-promoting and supportive of self-worth and the ability to accept oneself.

Spiritual level

It is often said by many people that pink is the colour of 'unconditional love'. This type of love is difficult for most humans to express if they are really honest with themselves. Compassion, however, takes into consideration our human frailties and foibles. Compassion is not weak. The red/white mix of pink shows the strength needed to be really compassionate. It takes a strong person to stand back and allow someone to learn to be who they are. Compassion isn't rushing in and trying to 'fix' everything or make it 'right', but it is the ability to offer freely all appropriate support. Compassion is accepting what 'is', with all the responsibility, pain and joy it can bring.

Summary: To increase or balance the pink energy in life

Wear a shade of pink you feel comfortable with.

Use pink crystals: rose quartz, rhodonite, rhodocrosite.

Use essential oils like rose, rose geranium.

Use flower essences of pink flowers: flowering currant, geranium, red campion etc.

Chakras: Linked to the sacral chakra and the heart chakra.

Brown

Brown is a mixture of red, yellow and blue. Like every colour, brown has a wide range of shades and tone, each having differing effects. It is primarily a colour of the earth and the natural world. Brown acts as a solid background colour, a base upon which other, more striking colours can arise. As a combination, brown is neutral and non-threatening. Its warm tones are comfortable and familiar.

The red content makes brown a colour of practical energy and this mixed with the mental qualities of yellow and blue can encourage study and focus of the mind. However, brown can also have a dulling effect in too large a quantity as it lacks the overall clarity to break out of established patterns of behaviour. Brown gives a state of solidity and reality from which one can grow. It suggests reliability and the desire to remain in the background, unnoticed.

Like black, it is associated with soil and the earth, though brown provides a safe environment for life free from the disturbing qualities that black can evoke. Brown encourages the practical expression of skills that take time to develop. The steady quality of brown ensures a thorough and accomplished outcome. Introducing brown into physical activity occurs through nature-based actions, like gardening, walking in woodland, crafting wood or working with clay. Wearing brown helps to keep stability and reminds us of the need to be practical.

Emotional level

All tones and shades of brown calm the emotions. In the view of ourselves, it can help us to feel more self-reliant. Like black, brown can also allow us to stay in the background and to remain detached from strong emotions. Brown is non-threatening when it is used as a main dress colour, as it can help the wearer to look more approachable and at the same time feel more secure. Chocolate is well known as a food that creates a feeling of well-being for many. Although thought of as a classic soother of emotions, too much can become addictive. Other brown foods, like nuts, can provide the same nutrients to stabilise the emotions without the short-lived buzz of sugar and cocoa. Hazelnuts are rich in the nutrients that help the pathways in the brain to function well, ideal for periods of thought or study.

Mental level

Brown is an excellent choice for surroundings involved with long-term study or logical thought processes. It helps ideas to become real, so it is very useful for the library or study of the visionary or inventor. Without the addition of daylight, brown can eventually dull the flow of original thought as it can create a strong need for stability and a love of routine. Brown can be used to help create new routines.

Spiritual level

On a spiritual level, brown shows the ability to integrate with one's surroundings. This encourages us to be content with where we are and with who we are, free from unrealistic wishes. This type of integration takes time, patience and effort. Like the primary colour components that create brown, this integration will represent all facets of the life and personality.

Summary: To increase or balance the brown energy in life

Wear brown clothes.

Use wood furniture in your home.

Eat brown foods (nuts, brown rice, seeds).

Use brown crystals: tiger's eye, dark citrine, staurolite, iron quartz.

Activities: walking, gardening, pottery, woodworking.

Chakra: Linked to the sacral chakra.

Grey

Grey is the true neutral colour. It is usually thought of as a combination of white and black, but the mixture of any complementary colours will produce grey. Grey is the colour of void, of emptiness, lack of movement, lack of emotion, lack of warmth, in fact, lack of any identifying characteristics. Because of this, grey can be restful. If it contains a high proportion of white it will tend to take on the qualities of surrounding colours. If the grey, though, has a greater amount of black, it can feel very heavy and depressing. Grey has a lack of information that has a numbing effect on the mind, though not particularly in a peaceful way, as blue or indigo might have. Indeed, the inability to see into the colour grey can be reminiscent of the experience of fear or terror where decision-making processes seem frozen and even time stands still. Emptiness, boredom, lack of direction, enervating and draining: the neutrality of grey prevents us from moving towards any energetic state.

Grey has no connection to the solid earth or the life of nature. Immovable stone and cloudy skies reflect the impersonal, implacable nature of grey. Grey has a detached, isolated and unemotional effect. Grey is a cool, calculating mental neutrality, an unwillingness to get one's hands dirty.

Grey can suggest someone who wishes to remain unsullied or uninvolved, but at the same time can suggest sophistication – being 'cool'. Indeed, when placed next to other colours, grey has the effect of moderating and stabilising those colours – both making them more visually apparent whilst muting the vibrational energy.

Grey clothes are still the favoured uniform of managers, businessmen and politicians reflecting the desire to project coolness of mind, emotional stability and the ability to look down on the rest of the world with detached neutrality – the epitome of the myth of efficiency.

Chakra: linked to the throat chakra.

Element: linked to space.

Working with colour and essences

The colour of a flower, plant, item or place can be linked to the matching chakra colour. Yellow flowers and gemstones would, in this way, be linked to the solar plexus chakra in the rainbow system and to the root chakra in the Vedic system. Essences of these would be useful when dealing with solar plexus chakra issues.

Sometimes the links are not so direct. A flower, plant, item or place can be matched to the correspondences of a colour that is different from its actual colour, when the effects of the essence are known. For example, yellow primrose works in a very 'red' way. It will have an effect on the solar plexus chakra from its yellow colour, but the energy it imparts has a lot of links to the root chakra and the colour red. It is helpful to code the essences available for use by colour, chakra, five-element and subtle body. Some producers already have this information in their essence catalogues.

Each colour has a complementary which, like the *yin/yang* symbol, balances any over-energy of that colour.

There are two systems of complementary colours too!

The 'True Colour' Complementary links are:

> Red – Turquoise
>
> Orange – Blue
>
> Yellow – Indigo
>
> Green – Magenta

These derive from colour as light.

The 'Artist's Wheel' Complementary links are:

> Red – Green
>
> Orange – Blue
>
> Yellow – Violet

These derive from colour as pigment.

From a chakra viewpoint the 'Artist's Wheel' complementary colours are also useful as they reflect the balancing relationship between certain chakras.

Working with issues to do with the root chakra has an effect on the heart chakra and vice versa. Working with the sacral chakra has an effect on the throat chakra and vice versa. Working on the solar plexus chakra has an effect on the brown and crown chakras and vice versa. For example, not only do yellow essences work well with solar plexus chakra issues, but so do indigo and violet vibration essences.

The advantages of using colour are that it is a language that bodies react to instinctively and clients can immediately appreciate the changes that colour elicits in them.

The disadvantages of using colour are that to work successfully with essences and colour, the colour correspondences need to be known well enough for the logical mind to begin assessment of appropriate essences and then for intuition, dowsing or muscle testing to continue.

However useful these correspondences may be, any colour can work with any chakra. Logical limitations should not therefore be placed on colour correspondences when intuition or assessment dictate otherwise.

CHAPTER 12

Protecting Personal Energy Integrity

Working in any setting where two or more people are interacting with each other can lead to inappropriate or inadvertent sharing or taking of someone else's energy. This can happen in everyday situations within the family, at work and in social interactions and is part of normal behaviour.

Within a therapy situation it is something to be aware of and to be avoided wherever possible. The therapist's role is to listen, support and make suggestions in order to help the client reach the outcome they seek. It is not helpful for the therapist to become entangled in the client's issues or problems.

There are several strategies to help to guard against inappropriate or inadvertent interactions.

Know thyself

Most practitioners have a need to be practitioners. Periods of inner reflection and silence are needed to discover why this role for helping others has been adopted.

There are classic scenarios that give rise to complementary and alternative practitioners ranging from personal illness, dysfunctional families to poor self-worth. Know and understand what the personal drives are!

Grounding

These days we often face the choice between a 'spiritual' life and a 'material' point of view. The new spirituality exhorts us to delve into the fine layers of existence, supposing that the more subtle energies that we know about, the better and more spiritual we will be. The problem is often that this tends to steer people away from the practicalities of living in the world, making it seem boring and lacking in glamour, or, as in many established religions, making it seem like some clever trap to prevent us from reaching spiritual goals. There are other views, however, that encourage us to fully engage with our lives and to embrace the world and its solidity. They tend to favour another mystical approach, believing that to really become who we are, we do indeed need to fully embrace our physical existence. For if our physical bodies are the focus point of all levels of our being, then it follows that we already have access to all the knowledge of the fine levels, even though we may not know it in ordinary awareness. What we don't have, these philosophies argue, is a solid experience of physical manifestation. To develop our full potential, therefore, we need to be 'here' and 'now'. Our focus needs to be both inward and downward. Inward to fully engage with the centre of our physical presence, and downward to link into the centre of our world.

It is very easy in the information-heavy world of the 21st century to place a huge amount of personal focus on ideas and fluctuating emotions. These often have tenuous links to the physical body and practicality. A lot of effort is then put into maintaining the ideas which have no firm basis in reality. This is a familiar stance taken in politics. Only by being grounded and in the 'now' can we resist being manipulated by others.

If we focus too much on the development of subtle skills and the knowledge of subtle energies without balancing them out by caring for the physical body and the development of our practical skills, then the energy balance in the body can easily be upset. The aura becomes top-heavy, with energy concentrated in the upper body and head, leaving little to feed the digestive system, reproductive system and lower limbs. Eventually these areas develop dysfunctions as they suffer from a continual lack of life-energy. This situation is common in urban societies where intellectual knowledge is valued above all other things.

The planet Earth is our main source of nurturing energy. It also provides a safe release point for excess or unwanted energy. These links to the planet are therefore crucial for our health and well-being.

Grounding is a common term used for the ability to maintain an energy connection to the planet. Grounding techniques can be divided into two types – passive and active.

Passive techniques

Passive techniques cover those actions that once completed, do not need further mental focus or reminding for them to stay effective.

Essences that are linked to certain crystals, most trees and specific environments can be used in drop or spray form to help to ground energies. Essences in the form of images or symbols can be carried without any further thought or attention.

Carrying crystals is a simple grounding technique. Ideal crystals for these processes are any dark coloured stones: red, brown, black and any metallic stones, as they naturally tend to stabilise, integrate and ground energies. If the stones have natural faceted terminations, ensure that they point down the body (towards the feet or ground) as this will emphasise their grounding and integrating qualities. Any use of crystals requires those crystals to be cleansed regularly by washing under running water, being passed through incense or smudge or sprayed with a cleansing spray.

Activities like drumming, dancing and strong physical exercise also have a grounding effect.

Eating sweet foods and food that are rich in protein can help the body to stay grounded.

Active techniques

Active techniques are those actions that need mental focus to stay effective. If someone is very ungrounded these are likely to be less effective as the nature of 'ungroundedness' often results in poor ability to concentrate and increased confusion.

Visualisations are the most common techniques employed. The simplest of these is visualising a thread of energy from the coccyx flowing down into the centre of the planet.

Mantras or other use of sound and vibration have been used for millennia to ground and protect personal energy. To be most effective the user needs to be very familiar with the sounds or words used. In many traditions there is a distinction made between mantras that can be used freely by all and those that require a specific transmission from an authorised teacher in order to be safe and effective.

Centring

This is a popular term for maintaining the central core of energy within the spinal axis of the body, ensuring that the body's energy is balanced. Centring techniques fall into the two categories of passive and active.

Passive technique: Carrying or wearing crystals

Wearing crystals on the centre-line of the body is an effective, passive centring technique. Apart from the red, brown, black and any metallic stones that are also grounding, fluorite and sugilite can be very useful. Crystals with striations, like topaz, aquamarine, kunzite and danburite are also very useful.

Active technique: 'Tapping in'

Tapping in (also described in Chapter 6) is one of the best active techniques for centring and steadying personal energies. To be most effective it should be practised every day, several times a day, until it becomes second nature.

It is also a useful technique before undertaking any form of energy or healing work. It not only protects from disruptive energies nearby and from other factors that may distract from work, but it also helps to ensure that any negativities from the therapist's energy field do not affect others. Most importantly, it also reduces the likelihood of the therapists absorbing negative energies from the client.

It is a very useful technique to do when there is frustration, nervousness or a need to recover from sudden shocks. The core of this technique is the tapping of the fingertips around the thymus area (top of chest).

This technique is also useful before beginning any dowsing or muscle testing, anchoring personal energies and thereby helping the dowsing or muscle testing to be more accurate. By centring your energies, the conscious mind is less likely to interfere with the results of the process.

'Tapping in' brings into balance all the major energy meridians of the body for about 20 minutes. It is also one of the simplest and most effective techniques for ensuring that a stable, centred energy is kept in place.

1. The simplest variation is a firm, light tapping with the fingertips on the area of the upper chest just below where the collarbones (clavicles) meet the breastbone (sternum). This is the approximate placement of the thymus gland, which is an important maintainer of the subtle energy balance in the body.

2. Whilst the thymus is being tapped, the other hand is placed palm open, over the navel. This allows the balancing effect to be longer lasting.

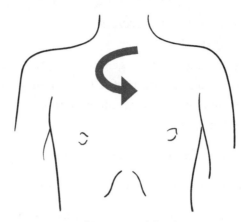

FIGURE 12.1 Placement of the thymus gland

3. Another variation of 'tapping in' is to tap anticlockwise (looking down onto the chest) in a circle about 8–15 cm away from the thymus point. Each tap of the fingers should be about 3 cm apart. Repeat the circle about 20 times.

4. Many important meridian channels pass close to the navel. Tapping around the navel about 8–10 cm away, this time in a clockwise direction, also has a balancing and centring effect.

5. Another variation of 'tapping in' is to tap anticlockwise (as you are looking down on your own chest) in a circle about 8–15 cm away from the thymus point. Each tap of the fingers should be about 3 cm apart. Repeat the circle about 20 times.

6. Many important meridian channels pass close to the navel. Tapping around the navel about 8–10 cm away in a clockwise direction also has a balancing and centring effect.

Tapping in should become an almost automatic process – a first step to ensure focus and accuracy before any therapy work is begun. The more familiar the body systems become to existing in a state of harmonious balance, the easier it is to maintain that balance and the more apparent it becomes when we occasionally lose that balance, ensuring that we notice and correct imbalances the sooner.

Centring and integrating exercises
1. COOK'S HOOK-UP

'Cook's hook-up' is excellent for general integration, co-ordination and grounding. It can also be useful when attention is starting to wander and the mind begins to meander off topic.

(Right-handed people)

a. Cross your ankles, right ankle over left.

b. Cross your wrists in front of you, right over left.

c. Rotate the wrists, so that the fingers fall downwards.

d. Interlace your fingers, and lay your hands on your lap.

e. Relax, close your eyes and breathe slowly.

f. After 2–3 minutes, release your hands and uncross your ankles.

g. Place your feet flat on the floor and rest the hands in your lap, with fingers spread.

h. Allow the fingertips of each hand to touch for a minute (as if you were holding a grapefruit between your palms).

If the person is left-handed, the left ankle and left hand are crossed over the right and so on for all directions.

2. EAR ROLLS

'Ear rolls' are useful when attention needs to be focused or thinking has become confused.

Beginning at the top of both ears (left fingers on left ear, right fingers on right). Using thumb and forefinger 'unroll' the outer edge of the ears and gently pull downwards, stretching the ear, working slowly down the lobes. Repeat three times.

3. CROSS CRAWL

'Cross crawl' is excellent for general integration, co-ordination and grounding. It can also be used to 'fix' affirmations into the whole body by repeating the affirmation whilst doing 'cross-crawl'. This can be done seated or standing – standing is better.

    a.   Lift the left knee a little, touching it with the right palm.

    b.   Then lift the right knee, touching it with the left palm.

    c.   Let your arms swing naturally and build up a natural rhythm.

    d.   Repeat about 20 times.

    e.   It can be done with the eyes closed.

Interpersonal behaviour

One of the most easily recognisable patterns in human behaviour is that described by the 'Karpman drama triangle' or the 'deadly triangle', as it has become known. Practitioners and healers are easily caught in this pattern, partly because of the intrinsic needs to be helpful to others but also because clients often see the practitioner as some sort of 'Rescuer'. Indeed some therapists see their clients as 'Victims'!

The only way to prevent this pattern developing is vigilance and a need for some deep personal reflection to understand what created the personal drive to be a practitioner in the first place. If there is an unconditional need to be the 'Rescuer' this needs to be looked at and dealt with.

The 'Karpman drama triangle' aka the 'deadly triangle'

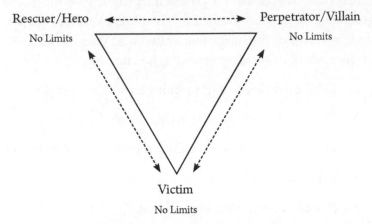

FIGURE 12.2 Drama triangle

There are three possible roles – 'Rescuer', 'Persecutor' and 'Victim'. In everyday language these could be renamed as 'Hero', 'Villain' and 'Victim'.

The 'Victim' always initiates the drama cycle. Once someone sees themselves as a Victim, someone else automatically fills the role of Persecutor/Villain. They fulfil the need for the Victim to blame.

The Victim may then begin to look for someone to act as a Rescuer/Hero. When these three roles are played out without any party holding their personal boundaries the 'drama triangle' becomes activated.

When activated, the Rescuer/Hero may help out without placing any limits on their aid. Eventually the Rescuer/Hero has to draw a limit as the Victim demands more and more of their attention and time. The Victim will then blame the Rescuer/Hero (who is now a Villain in the eyes of the Victim) for not being good enough, for failing them, for being part of the problem or something similar. The Victim will then have to look for another Rescuer/Hero.

In the meantime the original Perpetrator/Villain may be feeling like a Victim and start to look for their own Rescuer/Hero or someone to blame.

The original Rescuer/Hero would find themselves a Victim of the negativity and gossip of the original Victim and may start to blame that person or indeed might look for someone to come to act as a Rescuer/Hero.

In this way the drama triangle is self-perpetuating, self-escalating and very damaging.

The drama triangle is also very addictive. The emotional benefits can appear on the surface to be very empowering for the Victim. However, on closer inspection the power gain is from manipulation and misuse that needs constant feeding and only ceases when some responsibility is taken by the Victim for the situation they are in.

Even the most seasoned of practitioners will find themselves in a Karpman drama triangle; immunity against it does not exist. The knack as a practitioner, is to spot the beginning of the process of being pinned onto the drama triangle by a client and to prevent the process from gaining momentum.

Stopping the drama triangle is achieved by any one in the three roles keeping their personal boundaries firm and taking responsibility for situations. Others experiencing the drama triangle can then be encouraged to do the same.

A key point to remember is that everyone involved in a drama triangle will be trying to manoeuvre themselves into the role of Victim – this is the role where everything is everyone else's fault, and where the Victim believes they have done nothing inappropriate to warrant such treatment! Emotional investment in one's own point of view over those of others, and emotional responses – usually automatic and defensive – are what drives the drama triangle in all three of its roles.

Practical ideas to stop the process developing or escalation from a practitioner viewpoint are:

- Not being available 24/7.

- Having a dedicated practice phone/mobile with an answer machine.

- Saying a conditional 'Yes...but' or 'Maybe next week'.

- Getting into a routine for collecting clients' fees, maybe collecting money before the session.

- Saying 'Need to give that some thought...', don't agree to anything on the spot.

A practitioner should always work and relate to clients *within limits, within boundaries.* The practitioner must learn to stand back, give appropriate advice, but never 'bail out' the client from their responsibility to care for their own well-being. It is imperative that individual practitioners have enough personal awareness to prevent this powerful psychological game from gaining any momentum.

The drama triangle can be seen anywhere, but it is easy to identify within families and in the workplace. A person, family, company or other group of people have the capacity to occupy more than one place on the drama triangle.

Examples abound in the life of a practitioner; here is one:

Pippa is an excellent practitioner who is very sensitive to others' suffering and always willing to help. Mrs A came to see Pippa about the difficulties she was having with family and feelings of depression. It transpired that Mrs A felt she was being manipulated by her daughter into moving house. Mrs A eventually went away with an essence combination to help her deal with the situation. Mrs A settled the bill with Pippa, made another appointment in a few weeks and all was well.

In a few weeks Mrs A phoned to say she could not make the appointment in an hour's time and would Pippa make up another essence combination for her to use immediately. Pippa pointed out that she would still have to charge Mrs A for the appointment as the cancellation was too late for another client to take the slot, and taking the combination to Mrs A's house would involve fuel and time, so there would be extra for that. Pippa made up the combination and drove to Mrs A's house to deliver it. When Mrs A answered the door and Pippa offered the combination, she told Mrs A what the charge would be, but Mrs A refused to pay. Pippa pointed out politely that the cost had been agreed, but before Mrs A could answer Mrs A's daughter also came to the door. She shouted at Pippa, berating her for undermining her relationship with her mother and telling Pippa she was going to report her to the practitioner body for being unprofessional and over-charging. This the daughter did.

Fortunately Pippa had good client records and had a published policy of late cancellation. The practitioner body also had a fully functional complaints procedure.

Findings

A drama triangle was probably already running within the family. The visit to Pippa started to set up another with Mrs A as Victim, Pippa as Rescuer/Hero and the daughter as Perpetrator/Villain. Investigation from the practitioner body (the daughter's potential Rescuer/Hero) showed that the essence combination probably helped as the dynamics between the mother and daughter shifted. The mother had tried to put in some boundaries which made her less malleable and open to manipulation. By the second planned visit the drama triangle within the family had begun to escalate as the daughter realised that she was not going to get her way. The practitioner body suggested to Pippa that she might have considered posting the combination after payment had been received as that would have kept Pippa's boundaries firm and would have dissolved the new drama triangle being created in her practice. Pippa's eagerness to be too helpful had turned her from being the Rescuer/Hero (mother's viewpoint) into the Perpetrator/Villain (mother and daughter's viewpoint) and to a Victim (from the practitioner body's viewpoint). The practitioner body could find no 'fault' with Pippa's behaviour, so no disciplinary action was taken. Pippa never got the money for the combination. It was noted, however, that a few months later Mrs A had moved house.

There is a wonderful quote from the film *War Games* (1983) where David Lightman, a young hacker unwittingly accesses 'Joshua', a United States military supercomputer programmed to predict possible outcomes of nuclear war. 'Joshua' activates the countdown to nuclear missile release. During the ensuing drama Lightman manages to hack into the computer and get it to play tic-tac-toe (noughts and crosses) against itself. As a result the computer concludes that nuclear warfare is 'a strange game' in which 'the only winning move is not to play' – the same can be said of being involved with a Karpman drama triangle!

There are brilliant videos on YouTube about this drama triangle – please watch them!

Saying 'no' to treating a client

As an independent practitioner there is no obligation to treat any client. This applies to anyone regardless of who else has given consent – the client, the parent, or a medical professional.

If for any reason, a practitioner feels uneasy about treating someone, the practitioner can refuse to treat them and should never feel obliged to give a reason.

A client may be in a situation that creates discomfort for the practitioner in some way:

- the client may be a child

- the client may be pregnant

- the client may be suffering from physical, emotional or mental problems that the practitioner feels unable to work with

- the client may already be known to the practitioner

- the client may need palliative or end of life care

- the practitioner might feel unsafe with that client.

The key here is that if the practitioner feels in any way uneasy then their perceptive skills, empathic skills and clarity of thought will be compromised. It is up to the practitioner to identify their own personal issues and respect the boundaries and limitations they represent.

Getting support

A practitioner, no matter how busy a practice they have, needs to have people to go to or techniques to employ that support themselves in their work.

It is a good idea to get to know other practitioners with different skills in the locality. Trying out different therapies helps to broaden the personal approach, but also gives opportunities to get to know to whom clients might be able to be referred, where necessary.

Finding a practitioner of a therapy that is unfamiliar can be useful for personal well-being. Practitioners are notorious for being difficult clients. This is not usually because of their attitude, but often because their bodies 'know all the tricks in the book' and can be strongly protective, evasive and persistently stubborn when it comes to integrating their own healing.

It is also useful to find someone who can act as a mentor or a clinical supervisor. These would ideally be people who are experienced as practitioners, possibly also counsellors, who can listen and where necessary intervene and interact. Having someone to listen to the difficulties of dealing with clients and the issues that can arise within the practitioner as a result, can help maintain the well-being of the practitioner.

Another option is having peer group support from regular meetings with other practitioners. Cases can be brought to these types of sessions as long as they are kept anonymous and no information is shared that could identify clients. These are very important when dealing with situations where a client cannot be helped or where the Karpman drama triangle has been activated.

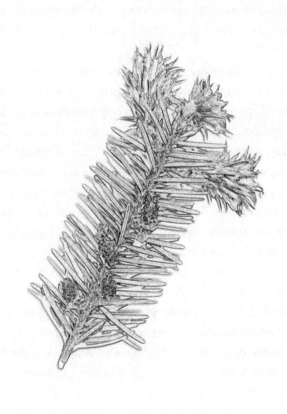

PART THREE

PROFESSIONAL PRACTICE

CHAPTER 13

CLIENT CARE AND MANAGEMENT

Client care and management is an integral part of being a professional practitioner, no matter what skill is used. The use of essences as a therapeutic tool is becoming more widely accepted and good practice by the essence therapist will support this expansion.

Guidelines quoted here are from UK and EU law, which is likely to be similar to those held by other countries worldwide.

The behaviour of a professional practitioner will be covered by a Code of Conduct linked to a practitioner association or come from the tutor that the practitioner trained with. If neither are available, the one held by the British Flower and Vibrational Essences Association is an excellent guideline.[1]

The following appear in most Codes of Conduct:

- Always maintain professional confidentiality regarding client's cases. Even in discussions with fellow practitioners refrain from naming names and giving details. Outlining general issues can be useful if support, supervision or mentoring is needed.

- Avoid criticising or finding fault with the work of a fellow practitioner or any member of the medical profession. Most Codes of Conduct state clearly that no matter what the

---

1   www.bfvea.com/downloadable-files.php, accessed on 27 July 2014.

situation, guidance given by a medical professional should not be countermanded. If a difficult situation arises then judicial use of language may be required. For example, if the issue of hormone replacement therapy is being discussed do not be drawn into giving personal opinions. People can always be directed to the internet if they want more information or another point of view.

Criticising the work or attitudes of other complementary and alternative practitioners has a tendency to backfire as people gossip. Better to have firm rules about being non-committal rather than give any opinion about anyone else's skill. However, it is useful to have a list of practitioners who are tried and trusted so that you can refer people where necessary.

- If a client is having current treatment for the same condition elsewhere, encourage the client to ask the medical or healthcare professional if they have any objections to the client receiving essences. It is always polite to suggest this to clients and make a note on the case history that you have done so. In practice few clients will ask or tell another practitioner that they are having treatment elsewhere.

- Never recommend that a client discontinue any drugs he or she may be taking. The decision must be taken by the client and their general medical practitioner. It might be very tempting to give an opinion in some situations and for many reasons. The temptation must be avoided. If necessary suggest the client talks things over with their general medical practitioner.

- Never diagnose or offer cures for specific conditions. In the UK it is against the law to 'diagnose' or to offer 'cures' unless qualified to do so. Practitioners assess and then suggest potential ways that the client can be helped. Do not even be tempted to use medical terminology like 'diagnosis'.

- Confine treatment to the particular skill or therapies that qualifications are held for. These will be the skills where there is up-to-date insurance to practice.

- Refer a client to another therapist or their general medical practitioner if it is felt that it is appropriate. Keep a written note of all recommendations to the client as exactly word-for-word as possible.

- Know personal limits and stick to boundaries.

- Appearance is important. As an essence practitioner a specific dress code (tunic, over-shirt, tabard etc.) is not needed but appearance should be neat and tidy. Be flexible in your appearance depending on where the practice is and try to avoid projecting any stereotype. Make sure that there is no possibility of being mistaken for a medical professional (dressing all in white or having a white overcoat). Try to avoid wearing too much jewellery.

- Always wash hands or use a disinfectant gel before and after the client session. Energetic cleansing of the workspace might also be an option.

- Keep to the timetable to ensure that subsequent clients are not kept waiting. This is professional, respectful and helps to build a firm financial base for the business.

The consultation

The consultation is extremely important as this is when decisions are made on the client's needs and suitability for treatment. During the time spent in the consultation several clues can help to identify the needs of the client and their expectations.

The tools at the practitioner's disposal are observation, asking questions and above all listening. If a professional association has not provided a case history form, then a practitioner can design one to suit their needs. Some practitioners request that a client completes a brief questionnaire before the first consultation; others have a simple format of questioning. A case history of some sort needs to be completed at a first session. Further case notes are then added to this that include essences suggested, frequency and length of time of use. The minimum required is usually the name, address or contact details and the name of the personal general medical practitioner. Date of birth should be included where relevant. A disclaimer that is signed by the client can be added to this, something on the lines of:

> I appreciate that flower and vibrational essence practitioners do not give medical diagnosis or treatment.
>
> I understand that my GP is medically responsible for me and my dependants.
>
> Signed: Date:

It is a good idea to remember, as with any notes made, that the client has the right to see them. Some practitioners actually get the client to sign the notes at the end of each session to confirm they are a true record and that they have had access to them. This is good practice.

Unlike some more physical therapies, working with essences does not require a detailed case history. After welcoming the client and helping them to feel at ease it is a good idea to explain about essences and enquire as to what has brought the client to the session.

Allow the client time to explain what is happening to them and make sure that everything is listened to. Ask questions where necessary and appropriate and record any relevant information onto the case history sheet.

Any suggestions made by the practitioner must be recorded in the case history. This protects the practitioner should any problem arise, but also lays the foundation for how the work might progress in subsequent visits. All records must be kept confidential.

It is good practice to complete the case history notes accurately at the time. If necessary the notes could be completed as soon as possible afterwards, but the client would then not be able to sign them as an accurate record of the session. The date should be added and preferably the time too.

If errors have occurred the practitioner should put a line through that information; it should be initialled and then the correct information written down. This is for clarity and transparency.

The Data Protection Act 1988

This Act requires that all personal data be protected. Even if the information is just a list of names and addresses, a business needs to be registered with the Data Protection Register.

It costs very little to be registered under this Act. Be sure to apply directly to the Information Commissioner's Office as third party companies will charge more than the annual fee.

- All information of a personal nature should be obtained and processed lawfully and fairly.

- Information should be held solely for treatment-specified reasons.

- Use information only for those purposes and disclose it only to people who have a legal right to it.

- Only hold data that are adequate and relevant.

The practitioner should reassure any client that registration under this Act has been done. In this way they can be assured that their contact details will not be passed onto anyone else.

Sale of Goods Act 1979 – The Supply of Goods and Services Act 1982

These two Acts cover the provision of essences and the act of the essence consultation.

This legislation identifies the contract of sale, which takes place between the retailer and the client/customer.

Both the above Acts cover consumer rights including goods being of merchantable quality, the conditions under which goods may be returned after purchase and whether goods are fit for their intended purpose.

A client disappointed with an essence consultation could take action against the practitioner if it were proved that reasonable care had not been taken under the terms of the Supply of Goods and Services Act.

- Keep all literature up to date.

- Be wary of making unrealistic claims that cannot be substantiated.

Trade Description Act 1968 and The Department for Business, Enterprise and Regulatory Reform (BERR) Office of Fair Trading Guidance

This Trades Act prohibits the use of false descriptions or to sell or offer the sale of goods which have been described falsely. BERR and the Office of Fair Trading cover situations when advertising or marketing has been misleading.

This covers advertisements such as oral descriptions and display cards. It applies to quality and quantity as well as to fitness for purpose and price. This also covers websites and social media.

It is important to understand that where an unsuitable description of an essence is given and repeated, the practitioner is equally as liable as the producer.

This Act is in conjunction with The Supply of Goods and Services Act 1982 and comes under the purview of the Advertising Standards Agency (ASA).

Advertising the practice

The MHRA Guidelines (Chapter 16) make it very clear how carefully words need to be chosen when advertising skills.

In addition to the MHRA there is a non-governmental body called the Advertising Standards Agency (ASA) that has taken to active policing of the complementary and alternative therapy scene in the UK.

If the MHRA Guidelines and the Code of Conduct information are followed and care is taken not to make any claims to cure or diagnose, advertising should not attract the unwelcome attention of the ASA. The ASA themselves do not have any legal powers as such, but can refer cases to Trading Standards who can act.

Treating children under the age of 18

It is illegal to give treatment to persons under the age of 18 without obtaining permission, preferably in writing from a parent or guardian prior to the treatment. A person over the age of 16 years and under 18 years may request medical attention by themselves. An essence practitioner is not recognised as a qualified medical practitioner, so if it is known that medical attention for the child is not being received, practitioners are advised to secure the signature of the parent or guardian to the following statement:

> I have been notified by _____ that according to law I should consult a doctor concerning the health of my child _____ (name of child).
>
> Signed _____ (parent or guardian).
>
> Signed by witness _____ (signature of person witnessing).

There is no legal minimum age at which a person can receive an essence from a practitioner. In the UK it is wise to ensure that as the practitioner, the Government Guidelines and Acts 1–3, which are concerned with the welfare and safety of children are followed.

If the child is of an appropriate age it should be established that they want to use essences on a voluntary basis, and that they have not been pushed into making a decision by an over-bearing parent or guardian. Should the child indicate they do not wish to have a consultation then the practitioner should not engage with the child under any circumstances. It is good practice to get written consent from the child where possible.

Parental or guardian consent is necessary. A child should not be examined or treated unless a parent or guardian is present or has given written permission and is present at the consultation. If the parent does not accompany the child to the consultation then written permission from that parent can be in the form of a letter.

However, it is good practice to never be alone with someone under the age of 16. For the protection of the practitioner an adult needs to witness the consultation at all times. If, for example, the parent(s) seems to be part of the problem, a chaperone can be suggested as the person present does not necessarily have to be the child's parent, but should be a responsible adult.

What must happen if it appears that the child is the victim of abuse

If the child discloses that they are being (or have been) abused, the practitioner has a moral and professional obligation to report this to the appropriate authorities.

If there are any doubts or concerns they should be reported to the NSPCC Child Protection Helpline for confidential advice on: 0808 800 5000.

The child should not be questioned by the practitioner. However, in the course of conversation the child may disclose the situation. Here it should be recorded and the report made later.

Criminal Records Bureau

Working with children or vulnerable adults may require registration with the Criminal Records Bureau (CRB). At present, self-employed practitioners are unable to apply for any level of Disclosure on a voluntary basis – though this will be possible when the CRB introduce the 'Basic Disclosure' service sometime in the future.

A self-employed person can apply for a DBS/CRB check by registering with an agency. The agency would be eligible to ask an exempted question as it would be the agency assessing the individual's suitability. In this example the agency could countersign the application form.

Specific disease-states

Notifiable diseases

It is a statutory requirement that certain infectious diseases are notified to the Medical Officer of Health of the district in which the client resides or in which he/she is living when the disease is diagnosed. The person responsible for notifying the Medical Officer of Health is the GP in charge of the case. If, therefore, a practitioner were to discover a notifiable disease that was clinically identifiable as such he should insist that a doctor is called in. Each local authority decides which diseases shall be notifiable in its area. There may therefore be local variations, but it is assumed that the following diseases are notifiable everywhere:

Acute encephalitis	Leprosy	Relapsing fever
Acute meningitis	Infective jaundice	Scarlet fever
Anthrax	Malaria	Tetanus
Acute	Leptospirosis	Tuberculosis
poliomyelitis	Measles	Typhoid fever
Cholera	Ophthalmia	Typhus
Diphtheria	neonatorum	Whooping cough
Dysentery	Paratyphoid fever	Yellow fever
Food poisoning	Plague	
Rubella	mumps	

Named diseases

UK law makes it an offence to take part in the publication of any advertisement referring to any article of any description in terms which are calculated to lead to the use of that article for the purpose of treating human beings for any of the following diseases: Bright's disease; glaucoma; cataract; locomotor ataxy; diabetes; paralysis; epilepsy or fits; tuberculosis.

It is also a criminal offence to publish any advertisement which:

a. Offers to treat or prescribe a remedy or advice for cancer, or

b. Refers to any article in terms calculated to lead to its use in the treatment of cancer.

The named diseases together with the words from the MHRA Guidelines in Chapter 16 make it very clear that any leaflets, websites or social media advertising a complementary or alternative practitioner must not be misleading or open to complaints.

Working with animals

In the UK the law on working with animals is very precise. The BFVEA negotiated and subsequently got clarification on how essences can be used with animals – from a practitioner's standpoint.

The law with regard to animal treatment is substantially more restrictive than for the treatment of human clients. The Veterinary Surgeons, in particular, Act 1966 (Section 19) provides, subject to a number of exceptions, that only registered members of The Royal College of Veterinary Surgeons may practise veterinary surgery. The latter is defined as encompassing:

The art and science of veterinary surgery and medicine and, without prejudice to the generality of the foregoing, shall be taken to include:

a. the diagnosis of diseases in, and injuries to, animals including tests performed on animals for diagnostic purposes

b. the giving of advice based upon such diagnosis

c. the medical or surgical treatment of animals and

d. the performance of surgical operations on animals [...]

The people who may legally administer *minor medical treatment* to an animal are:

- its owner

- another member of the household of which the owner is a member

- a person in the employment of the owner.

Additionally, any person may render emergency first aid to an animal 'for the purpose of saving life or relieving pain or suffering'.

Veterinary surgery involving acupuncture, homoeopathy and other complementary therapy may only be administered by a veterinary surgeon who should have undergone training in these procedures.

It is legal for essence practitioners to work with animals as long as they do not practise veterinary surgery or give medical treatment. They may, for example, provide animal owners or carers with essence treatments to support an animal's emotional and psychological well-being. They may also provide owners and carers with suggestions for applying or using such essences. Such practices remain legal as long as the essence practitioner:

- does not give a diagnosis of disease or injury in animals

- does not perform tests for the purpose of diagnosing physical disease or injury

- does not give medical advice based upon a medical diagnosis

- does not perform surgical operations

- does not supply anything which counts as a veterinary medicine for the purpose of Veterinary Medicines Regulations.

Using essences with animals

It is always wise for essence practitioners to ensure that animal owners have sought professional help from a veterinary surgeon for any problems the animal is experiencing.

Practitioners are, therefore, advised to secure the signature of the owner or keeper of such an animal to the following statement:

> I confirm that I have been notified by _____ (name of practitioner) that I should consult a veterinary surgeon regarding the health of my animal_____ (name of breed).
>
> Signed_____ (Owner/keeper of animal).
>
> Signed by witness_____ (Signature of person witnessing).

A very efficient way of introducing an essence to an animal is through the aura. The owner places a drop of the essence on one hand, rubs their hands together and then passes their hands through the aura or fur of the animal. This has the extra advantage of the owner also getting the benefit of the essence! Pets often take on the concerns of their owners and using essences this way helps to deal with both.

Working from a distance; absent work

Some practitioners are drawn to working with animals, people and places whilst not being personally present. This can be done over the phone, by email, Skype or by post.

If the client is not personally present, then permission and a 'witness' need to be obtained. This could be a signature, hair, astrological birth chart or photo. Assessment would then be carried out by dowsing or finger testing.

The advantages of working this way are:

- not having to have a clinic or practice space

- can work when needed, not tied to a timetable.

The disadvantages of working this way are:

- it is easy for personal energy to be compromised, care must be taken to 'disengage' from the client fully after the session

- it is harder to pitch the cost of the work undertaken and essences sent in the post

- it is harder to follow-up unless there is a firm routine and timescale.

Can someone 'block' the efficacy of an essence?

The short answer is 'Yes'.

There are at least two scenarios that occur when an essence(s) can seem to be blocked from working by the client.

The first scenario sometimes occurs when clients have very low prana/chi or may have some form of chronic fatigue. This sort of situation can also result in difficulties in processing other energy input, like homoeopathy, reiki and hands-on healing. The body's ability to process information can be extremely poor and so the body 'parks' the healing information or healing energy somewhere for use at a later date. Enthusiastic practitioners can inadvertently aggravate this by trying harder and harder. The key here is to do much less, in fact, maybe to offer a single essence to be taken or used in one drop, once a day. When the client's body becomes familiar with processing that one drop and indicates change, the process can move on.

The second scenario sometimes occurs in people who have very strong personal views about essences not being able to do anything, or indignity at being dragged along by a worried parent, guardian or partner to get an essence to help with a problem or issue.

> When teaching we explain the scenario like this: pharmaceuticals open a door for a client and kicks them through it whether they want to go or not. Homoeopathy and herbal products can also have this effect.

> With essences, though, open the door and leave the choice of whether the client goes through it or not, to the client and/or the client's body.

> Excerpt from *Plant Spirit Healing Workshops*,
> Simon and Sue Lilly, 1994–2014.

CHAPTER 14

METHODS OF MAKING ESSENCES

I do not, when making essences, communicate directly or perceive spirits, though they make themselves felt. I feel that the less I can be involved energetically, the better for the clarity and purity of the essence. The essence is, after all, of the plant, tree or whatever, not of me meditating, musing, daydreaming, chatting to or otherwise interacting with the plant. There is no way of avoiding some energy interaction, but I prefer to keep it to the minimum at the making stages.

Excerpt from *New Vibrational Flower Essences of Britain and Ireland*, Simon Lilly, edited by Rose Titchiner *et al.*, 1997.

The process of making an essence starts when the intention arises in the mind of the producer. Any events, coincidences or other significant thoughts and feelings should be noted from this point onwards. It is likely that the essence that will be made will reflect these in some way.

Many essence producers make a point of 'asking permission' to make an essence or attuning to the plant, item or environment before any action is begun.

Some essence producers stay close, meditate or attune to the focus of the essence in some way, during the time that the essence is being made. This too can help to determine or discern what the essence may be useful for.

Some producers decide to stay well away from the essence whilst it is being made to allow the focus of the essence to be to the sole influence.

Whichever stance is taken, it has become apparent from the work of Kröplin *et al.* (see Chapter 2) that the producer has an effect on the essence.

After the essence is first made the 'mother' essence, as it is called, is preserved in brandy or other alcohol. This helps to 'set' the energy of the essence into the water and preserves the water. Even if a non-alcoholic version of the essence is then made, alcohol is still the most efficient way of stabilising the 'mother'.

Making essences is a co-creative process with Nature. Making links with Nature in this way can also be quite addictive and creates quite a 'buzz'! Often once someone has made their first essence they will quickly look around for an opportunity to make others.

Method 1 – The boiling method

Eighteen of the traditional Bach Flower Remedies range are made by the 'boiling' method.

Here the flowers or parts of the plant should be freshly picked, preferably early in the morning and placed in a clean saucepan. There should be enough plant material for the saucepan to be three-quarters filled with the flower and twigs/stems. The flowers and twigs/stems should be covered with just over a litre of pure water and the mixture brought to the boil without the lid on. The mixture is then left to simmer for 30 minutes. The pan should then be removed from the heat source, the lid placed on the pan and left to cool outside, in the open air.

When the mixture is cold, the resulting water should be filtered through an unbleached filter paper (this is now the mother essence).

Method 2 – The sunlight method

This is the classic method by which 20 of the Bach Flower Remedies and many essences worldwide are made.

If flowers are the focus of the essence, they should be freshly picked early in the morning on a bright sunny day. The making of other types of essence should also begin early in the morning, if possible.

A thin glass bowl, which has no markings on it, is filled with pure water, preferably freshly drawn from a spring. Any plant material is then floated on the water surface. In most cases the surface of the water would be covered with plant material.

The bowl and its contents are then left in the sunshine for 3–4 hours. The plant material is then removed and the mother essence (the water that remains) is filtered through an unbleached filter paper to remove any plant material and poured into a bottle at least half full of brandy or other alcohol. The bottle should then be labelled with the name of the plant or other focus and the date the mother essence was made.

The other methods (other than boiling) follow this pattern. Nowadays many producers feel that unbroken sunlight is not necessary to create the shift in the water's energies. However, if a traditional Bach Flower Remedy range is being made, Dr Bach's protocol needs to be followed to the letter to be able to officially say the essences are 'made with the traditional methods described by Dr Edward Bach'.

Method 3 – Environmental essences

One of the Bach Flower Remedy range (Rock Water) is made by simply placing a bowl of spring water in sunshine.

Other environmental essences are made in a similar way by placing a bowl of spring water in sunshine or moonshine.

The mother essence (the water that remains) is filtered through an unbleached filter paper to remove any dust and poured into a bottle at least half full of brandy or other alcohol. The bottle should then be labelled with the name of the place or other focus and the date the mother essence was made. Any environmental essence for places, weather conditions or celestial events can be made in this way.

Method 4 – Flower essences – other methods

There are several variations for making flower essences that do not involve detaching the flowers from the plant.

- A bowl with water might be placed close to the plant with the intention of the water picking up the energy signature of the plant or by dripping water over the blooms and collecting the infused water. (This is useful for flowers that cannot be teased into dipping their blooms into the water without removing them or breaking the stems.) This is an indirect method.

- Some flowers' stems can be teased and bent using thin thread into dipping their living blooms into a bowl. If flowers are hanging downwards from a twig, a small jar with water could be suspended from the twig so that the living flower is under the water.

- A crystal might be programmed to collect the energy from a flower.

- The essence could be made at night, with or without moonlight. This is useful for plants that flower in the evening or if a more *Yin* essence is required.

The mother essence (the water that remains) is filtered through an unbleached filter paper to remove any dust and poured into a bottle at least half full of brandy or other alcohol. The bottle should then be labelled with the name of the place or other focus and the date the mother essence was made.

Method 5 – Mineral/gem/crystal essences

The mineral, crystal or gem will need to be energetically cleansed before making the essence. This can be done by any method in Appendix 2. The mineral, crystal or gem can then be placed in water *if it is safe to do so*. Some minerals can be toxic or soluble in water.

If there is any uncertainty, use one of these indirect methods:

- A bowl of water might be placed close to the mineral, crystal or gem, with the intention of the water picking up the item's energy signature.

- A 'bain-marie' set-up, with one small bowl inside another, can be used. The mineral, crystal or gem is then placed in the inner bowl and the water poured into the outer one.

The bowl of water can then be left in sunlight or moonlight.

The mother essence (the water that remains) is filtered through an unbleached filter paper to remove any dust and poured into a bottle at least half full of brandy or other alcohol. The bottle should then be labelled with the name of the mineral, crystal or gem and the date the mother essence was made.

In some countries all mineral, crystal or gem essences are required to be made by an indirect method for the essence to be sold.

Method 6 – Channelled essences (non-physical imprint)

This increasingly popular method of making essences requires the producer to more be directly involved.

- The producer is required to invite, evoke or invoke the presence or quality of a symbol, energy entity, animal, plant, emotional state etc. into the water to re-pattern it.

- The ability of the producer to focus on the target energy will qualify how well the water is re-patterned with the required energy. Some people may have a complex ritual for them to feel content with the essence produced. Other may act spontaneously. They key here is whatever it takes for the connection and communication to be made. There are no rules. If the connection made is not clear then the energy of the resulting essence will be confused.

Method 7 – Radionic or energy essences

These require specialist equipment and in some case extra training.

Use of radionic equipment to attract or copy the energy of specific items has been available for over a century. More recent equipment has given producers the opportunity to use sound and light recordings of plants, items or environments. Those producers drawn to these methods usually already have an interest or the necessary expertise.

The 'mother' essence

Once the 'mother' essence has been preserved many producers taste a small amount of the unpreserved mother essence. This can give a good idea of the quality of the essence and the water can taste very special. It is also an opportunity to acknowledge and thank the source of the essence. Any remaining mother essence is often returned to the plant or environment.

One or more drops of the mother essence are then diluted into another bottle to create a 'stock' dilution. Many essence producers sell essences at this dilution and it should say so on the bottle or in the literature from the producer. 'Stock bottles' are at the dilution that is most useful for practitioners. From stock dilutions, dosage bottles can be created for clients.

If one or more drops of stock essence are diluted into another bottle, this creates a 'dosage' bottle. Some producers sell at this level of dilution. It should say this on the bottle or in the producer's literature, though, unfortunately, this is not always the case. Dosage bottles are ideal for selling onto clients.

Setting up a workspace for making up essences

Guidelines quoted here are from UK and EU law which is likely to be similar to those held by other countries worldwide.

Essences are widely accepted as food and all rules and regulations for food hygiene are technically applicable. The only other two categories available in the UK are cosmetic and medicine. Both of these have their own sets of regulations.

Making essences with a permanent dedicated space

This is what should be aimed at in an ideal situation when there is a room that can be dedicated solely to essence production:

- An easily cleaned area made of plastic/Formica, NOT wood. Cleanable cupboards, washable walls, shelves and lino flooring. Ideally worktops and floors should be sealed. This is really like a normal kitchen.

- There must be two sinks, one for washing equipment and one for washing hands. These sinks need to be labelled. A bottle of antibacterial hand wash should be on hand. Double sinks have proved to be adequate.

- No animals should be allowed in the area, or outside coats or shoes.

- Overalls are advised as are plastic gloves and hair-coverings.

- Sterilising equipment.

- A liquid sanitiser (antibacterial surface wash), preferably biodegradable, may be advisable, although alcohol is quite good for this!

- Look out for courses at local colleges on food hygiene. These will give clear guidance on what should be done.

Making essences without a permanent dedicated space

The Women's Institute Markets in the UK have built up a very responsible position in the campaign for food safety. Their guidelines are ideal for those just beginning the process of making essences for sale, or for those who have a very small production with no permanent dedicated space.

These procedures would need to be followed *every* time essences are prepared. The points are as follows:

1. Environmental Health officers have the right to inspect premises without notice.

2. All involved must obtain a Basic Hygiene for Food Handlers certificate and attend the refresher course every three years.

3. In the room to be used there must be an overall atmosphere of cleanliness.

4. There should be an adequate supply of hot water, detergent, nailbrush and disposable towels, clean utensils and worktops.

5. Any pets and their bedding must be removed.

6. The room must be free from laundry and outerwear.

7. First aid materials must be readily available.

8. Thoroughly clean and disinfect all work surfaces using food-friendly cleaners.

PERSONAL INFORMATION

1. Have a professional attitude to personal cleanliness and know the risks of contamination.

2. No smoking.

3. Wear protective clothing and hair covering.

4. Do not prepare items when the producer or a member of the family is unwell, especially after a cold or stomach disorder.

5. Cuts or abrasions should be covered with a suitable dressing.

6. Hands should be thoroughly washed regularly.

FURTHER INFORMATION

UK Food Hygiene (General) Regulations 2006.

UK Food Safety Act 2006.

UK Bottling Guidelines

All essences are treated as foods whether they are intended for internal use or not. As such they are subject to food production laws (Health and Safety: Food Hygiene) and food labelling laws (UK DEFRA Regulations 1996. These are being superseded as new EU nutritional labelling is adopted from 2016).

If essences are being used in cosmetics or used with something that is not edible, then the product is a cosmetic and needs to be dealt with under cosmetic regulations (see page 222).

1. If essences are being made for sale to the public, or even if dosage bottles are being created a Basic Food Hygiene Certificate should be considered.

2. The site for bottling needs to comply with food guidelines.

3. The essence must be bacterially inactive. This can be achieved by sterilisation, proper handling and preservative. Some producers think that sterilisation may not be required if the alcohol content prevents bacterial growth. Alcohol content of over 20–22 per cent is absolutely essential to accommodate this point of view.

4. Basic personal hygiene and monitoring of the environment will ensure no contamination occurs.

5. Preservative – this has traditionally been brandy. Vodka, glycerol or vinegar are options but concentrations must be sufficient to prevent bacterial growth.

6. Tamper-evident bottles/bottle-tops are advisable when selling to the public.

7. Literature and advertising must comply with current laws and also comply with Medicines and Health Products Regulatory guidelines.

Hazard Analysis Critical Control Point (HACCP)

This is a well-established system of hazard analysis, which helps food businesses to ensure that everything that should happen in a workplace to protect food safety does indeed take place. It involves keeping records.

The principles of HACCP are:

- Assessing the potential food safety hazards in work activities.

- Identifying the points where hazards occur and deciding which are critical for food safety – these are the 'critical control points'.

- Implementing appropriate controls for eliminating or reducing each hazard.

- Establishing a monitoring system to ensure that the controls are effective – what should happen does happen.

- Setting up procedures to correct any problems.

- Reviewing the system from time to time and whenever operations change.

- Documenting the hazard analysis.

Most producers are 'one-person' operations, and as essence makers there are only a few instances where the essence could be contaminated. It is a good idea to look at the routine and identify those activities where contamination could happen and make a record of what is actually done.

As soon as your production involves more than one person, this procedure becomes VERY important!

An idea of what a HACCP plan could be for a small producer

- Record of each mother essence – common name, Latin name, date, place, method, how much made, photograph.

- Record of delivery of bottles –who, what, when, check for breakage.

- Record of delivery of brandy/vodka – who, what, when, batch number, visual check.

- Record of delivery of hydrosol – who, what, when, visual check.

- Record of each time the dedicated space is prepared.

- Record of each time essence bottles are sterilised – date, what size bottles, how many.

- Record of each time bottles are used with what percentage of preservative – date, what size, how many.

- Record of each stock produced – what essence, date, what size, who for, batch number, expiry date.

- Record of what is sent to whom.

It is a good idea to keep one 10 mL essence back from each batch as a record of stability, to be kept for seven to ten years.

More information on dilutions

Homoeopathic dilutions

Homoeopathic dilutions take the initial infusion of an item (liquid A). Dilutions are then made sequentially, taking one drop of the liquid into 1000 or more drops of water. This is then succussed (shaken vigorously thousands of times) – liquid B.

Drops of liquid B are then diluted and succussed again and then diluted and succussed again and again. Each dilution milestone is given a code.

1:100 = 1D (c or x) is when the procedure has been carried out 100 times.

1:1,000,000 = 6D (c or x) is when the procedure has been carried out a million times.

Succussing and dilution in this way changes the polarity of the liquid. This then acts on the body in a different way from simple dilutions. The resulting products tend to be experienced as more *Yang*, very energised.

Herbal dilutions

Herbal dilutions can be tisanes (teas), infusions (boiled, and left to soak or steep), decoctions (mashed and then boiled and cooled concentrations) or tinctures (alcoholic extractions). These are seldom diluted any further and therefore contain the active biological ingredients of the source.

The 'boiling method' of making essences initially makes a decoction of the plant materials. This may be why the essences in the Bach Flower Remedy range that have come from the boiling method have a little more 'kick' to them.

Essences

Essences have only one or two simple dilutions from the 'mother essence', most usually two. Up to seven drops of the 'mother essence' are placed into a small bottle (usually 10 mL or 30 mL) of brandy or other alcohol. This is usually then called a 'stock' bottle and is the item sold as an essence. Approximate dilution ranges from 1:100 to 1:500.

In essences there is no trace of the original item, even when made by the 'boiling method'.

So where plants are used which may appear on some notional list of 'potentially dangerous' herbs, by virtue of these standard methodologies, there is not a danger. It may be prudent to make essences from known toxic plants using an indirect method. However, even when toxins are found in one part of a plant, they may not be found in another. Alkaloids may be present in the green fruit but not in the flower. Reports of toxicity may be based upon ingestion of the root or bark, but not the leaves or buds.

For example, evidence is available from a chemical test searching for alkaloids that demonstrates the absence of alkaloids from cherry plum and elm essences where they might be otherwise expected.

Storing essences

Essences should be stored in such a way that bottles do not touch each other. This is especially important for mother essences. It ensures that the vibrational integrity of each mother essence is intact. Even stock dilutions benefit from being stored without contact for the same reason. Boxes can be obtained from suppliers or each bottle can be surrounded with cardboard.

Essences should be stored away from strong smells, electricity cables and equipment. Extremes of temperature should also be avoided and storage in darkness is best. Carefully looked-after essences maintain their integrity for many years.

Shipping or taking liquid essences from one country can be complex. Shipping requirements vary from place to place. Concern is always raised when taking essences in airline hand luggage or hold luggage as to going through X-rays and other checks.

Some people prefer to wrap essences in aluminium foil to help protect their essences. Others use a charging technique to clear any unwanted disruption to their essences.

Enhancing or charging essences

It has been suggested that essences can benefit from 'charging', that is, increasing their energy or enhancement in some way. This is a matter of personal choice and experimentation.

Essences can be 'charged' when they are first made and again each time the mother essence is disturbed.

Here are several methods – there may be others:

Method 1 – from the 1980s

In *Gem Elixirs and Vibrational Healing Vol. II* by Gurudas, it is suggested that one way of charging essences is to use a copper pyramid. This can be created by making a 60° angled four-sided pyramid of cardboard or of metal wire or tubing.

Do not recreate or buy a Cheops (Egyptian) pyramid that has an internal face-angle of about 52° as this creates a dead-space in the centre. Energy workers specialising in geopathic stress describe this area as being 'negative green' in its effect on human life by disrupting the life force.

HOW TO MAKE A SMALL PYRAMID AT
60 DEGREES, WIDTH OF EACH SIDE IS
6 INCHES, HEIGHT 8 INCHES

1. Using plant sticks, cut four pieces 6 inches long and eight pieces 8 inches long.

2. Take one of the 6-inch sections and two of the 8-inch sections.

3. Using masking tape or clear sticky tape, join them up to create a triangle. At the angles leave a gap between each piece of stick

to allow the joint to bend. The apex is a bit fiddly, but just do the best possible!

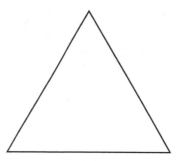

FIGURE 14.1 Create a triangle

4. Do this with all the pieces, giving four triangles in all.

5. Lay the triangles on a flat surface and begin joining them together with more tape, as in Figures 14.2 and 14.3

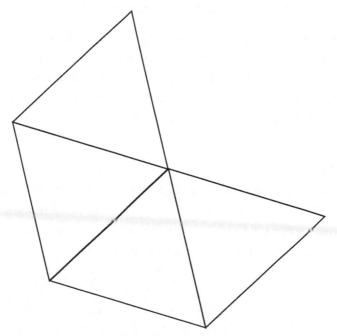

FIGURE 14.2 Join four triangles

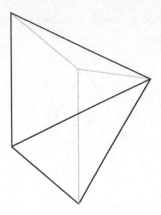

FIGURE 14.3 Form a pyramid

6. Join the last two uprights together to form a pyramid.

7. Using pliable copper wire, begin to wind the wire around each stick.

8. Mould the shape to hold its geometry.

The pyramid can be surrounded with crystals (clear quartz and lodestone) to add more energy. This pyramid is used by placing the essence(s) in the centre of the pyramid space and leaving it there for a few hours. A bigger pyramid can be created by increasing the length of the sticks in proportion to each other.

Method 2

There are special pendulums, a crystal pendulum or specific designs like an 'Isis' pendulum, that can 'charge' essences by rotating the pendulum above the essence (obtainable in several sizes from: www.emeraldinnovations.co.uk, accessed on 27 July 2014).

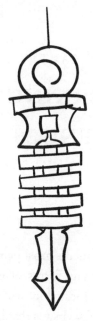

FIGURE 14.4 A pendulum

Method 3

Some producers use personal awareness and bless their essences, some use Reiki symbols, other symbols, mantras or prayers.

Method 4

'Light-Life Rings' have also been found to be very effective and easy to use (obtainable from www.lightlifetools.co.uk/Rings.htm, accessed on 27 July 2014).

CHAPTER 15

DISCERNING WHAT
ESSENCES 'DO'

Once essences have been made, most people are keen to know what an essence 'does'. Like many forms of energetic healing, how an essence interacts with an individual will be unique to that person. There are many books and websites that list essences and what they 'do'. Indeed it is difficult to sell essences to practitioners and the public without including a sentence or two of explanation.

Since essences have been in the 'foods' category, making medicinal or physical claims for essences without scientific proof is considered outside the law. A long, fruitless project could attempt to redefine what the nature of 'scientific proof' is, but there has been much useful work carried out from a subject viewpoint into the efficacy of essences.

Nevertheless it is a good idea for any practitioner to have their own methods of discerning what any essence 'does' regardless of what others have written about it. After all, a producer or author can only write so much about any one essence and there is always more to find out. If a practitioner is making their own essences then this type of assessment can be very useful.

This is one strategy that can provide a thumbnail sketch of what an essence 'does' from personal experience:

1. If an essence has just been made, take note of events that happened just before, during and after the making where this is appropriate.

2. Record the habitat, colour, qualities etc. of the source of the essence.

3. Draw a wide margin on the left-hand side of a sheet of paper and having taken or used that essence, record the following on the left:

   Using a pendulum or muscle/test:

   Which chakra the essence *mainly* works on?

   Which chakra(s) it works on physically?

   Which ones – emotionally, mentally, spiritually?

4. Which meridian(s) does the essence mainly work on?

5. Does the essence resonate to any particular subtle body?

6. Any other thoughts, images, dreams etc.

7. Record the experiences of 'tuning into' the plant or essence source.

If the skills are available to work with sonic driving (shamanic journeying) or similar techniques (see Gateway Visualisation, Appendix 5), record impressions and experiences.

When these have been ascertained and recorded on the left of the page, start to put a few words of comment on the findings, this time on the right-hand side of the sheet.

When ideas have been gathered, sit down and write a few sentences bringing the notes together. Pay particular attention to repeating images or patterns.

The essence can be offered to friends and colleagues and their responses collated with the primary assessment. The more people that feedback and experiences can be obtained from, the better the energy picture of that essence will be.

In this way a fuller picture of how an essence works can be obtained. For books, catalogues and websites the repeating patterns would be given emphasis so that practitioners and members of the public can see how the essence might affect the majority of users.

The following is an example of discerning an essence, courtesy of Steve Mason.

Record Sheet: Discerning the qualities of an essence

Name of essence: Lithium Quartz

Lithium (or Lithia) Quartz is clear quartz (SiO_2) with inclusions of lepidolite $(K(Li,Al)_3(Si,Al)_4 O_{10} (F,OH)_2$ or spodumene $(LiAlSi_2O_6)$. It tends to be violet or lavender in colour.

	Item	Findings	What this could indicate
1	Events when making or info about essence maker	I was feeling really fed up at this time and a bit stuck in a rut and also I think quite lonely and isolated.	I think I focused on making essences and working with crystals etc. as they made me feel better. This stone was most likely chosen as I felt depressed and thought it might help.
2	Habitat, colour etc.	Made using direct method on a rare sunny day in December. A peachy/brown colour stone with pale winter sun.	Hope, the promise of brighter days to come. A yearning for the summer and for sunlight to return to my life.
3	Main chakra?	Heart and pericardium.	Protects the heart and allows time to heal. However, it could also show a tendency to lock the heart and shut others out?
	Any on physical level?	It has a physically numbing effect, sort of disconnecting.	Not entirely unpleasant, it feels a bit like being sedated but it's very subtle. It feels like relaxing deeply into a hot bath and just zoning out.
	Emotional?	Elicits a feeling of detachment.	Releases anxiety or over-thinking; this may connect it to liver energy and a fixed attitude.
	Mental?	As above it calms the mind but also made me feel more able to focus and get things done.	Shifts an attitude of not being bothered and allows you to focus by moving beyond daily worries and anxiety.
	Spiritual?	By stilling and opening the mind it allows meditation to come more easily.	The mental disconnect allows deeper access to the subconscious.
4	Main meridian?	Spleen and liver.	Spleen as it is effected by anxiety. Liver, resentment and pent up emotions linked closely to anxiety need to be released or negative liver energy invades the spleen.
5	Other impressions?	Time out.	This isn't an 'end' essence; it's to be used as part of a plan of recovery. Could be used in cases of addiction or depression but it's a bit of a 'clean onsite rubbish' essence. Others, I feel, would need to be used after to rebuild layers of injury or feelings of loss etc.
6	Tuning in?	A sense of spiritual energy beyond time, space and above human worries and concerns.	Ascended spirits are beyond humanity, so don't share our worries though they are compassionate to our pain.
7	Core Shamanic link?	Journeys took me to a desert realm. It taught me that this is a tone/essence for those who are isolated or who feel they are having their metaphoric time out in the wastelands alone.	This stone/essence creates space when you need it, but detaching you emotionally and mentally. It can also act as a callback when it's time to start the long journey back to yourself.

CHAPTER 16

SELLING ESSENCES TO THE PUBLIC

Guidelines quoted here are from UK and EU law, which is likely to be similar to those held by other countries worldwide.

Labelling law

All essences are treated as foods whether they are intended for internal use or not. As such they are subject to food production laws (Health and Safety: Food Hygiene) and food labelling laws (UK DEFRA Regulations 1996. These are being superseded when EU nutritional labelling is adopted in 2016).

If essences are being used in cosmetics or used with something that is not edible, then the product is a cosmetic and needs to be dealt with under cosmetic regulations (see page 222).

The UK DEFRA Food Labelling Regulations 1996, Document 1499

a. The name of the food [to include what it is, i.e. essence etc.].

b. A list of ingredients [in descending order of volume or weight].

c. The appropriate durability indication [expiry date/best before date/use by, batch number].

d. Any special storage conditions or conditions of use.

e. The name or business name and an address [post code is OK, telephone number is not OK].
    – the manufacturer or packer or
    – the seller established within the EC.

f. Particulars of the place of origin or provenance, if failure to provide this could mislead.

g. Instructions for use [unless label is less than 10 cm² in which case this can be omitted].

From 2016, labels for containers with a surface exceeding 25 cm square will need to have nutritional information on them.

What can and can't be said about what an essence 'does'

Commercial essence producers, certainly those within the UK, are aware of what can be said and what should be avoided when it comes to describing what essences 'do'.

Producers and practitioners are strongly advised to avoid these words and phrases when describing essences or practitioners' work with essences as they may contribute to the MHRA determining that essences described with these words are **medicines** *and need the necessary licenses, premises and testing procedures.*

This list is not exhaustive:

Alleviates	Burns fat	Can lower cholesterol
At the first sign of…	Calm/calms/ calming	Clears
Avoids	Can benefit those who suffer from …	Clinical trials evidence
Boosts the immune system		Clinically proven

Combats

Controls

Counteracts

Cure/cures

Eliminates

Fights

Heals

Helps body adjust after crossing time zones

Help maintain a normal mood balance

Increases metabolic rate

Is said to help with...

Medical research...

Prevents/ preventing

Protects against

Remedies

Removes

Repairs

Restores

Stimulates the nervous system

Stops

Stops cravings for...

Strengthens the immune system

Strips off sun-damaged pre-cancerous cells

Traditionally used for

Treats/clears infestations

Treats/ treatment/ treating

Excerpt from MHRA Guidance Note 8 – With respect to words and phrases that the MHRA associate with medicines

This list from the MHRA is a minefield for people writing about essences. Although the words in themselves do not define 'medicines', it has to be borne in mind that essences usually come in little bottles and are often taken by mouth – like most medicines are.

When the essence is not a food

Many practitioners and producers use creams, roll-ons, sprays (that contain essences and essential oils) and other cosmetic vehicles for essences. Since the Cosmetic Law changed in July 2013, this is no longer a straightforward situation.[1]

Any base product that has been bought in must have been tested by the manufacturer and anything that is made and sold by them must have been tested by the seller.

> As a manufacturer or supplier you could be held liable in any legal action for harm caused to consumers or businesses as a result of unintended side-effects or the failure of products manufactured or supplied by you.
>
> From Department for Business, Innovation and Skills, 2012

---

1   www.gov.uk/product-safety-for-manufacturers, accessed on 27 July 2014.

DETAILS OF A SUNLIGHT/ WATER METHOD

1. Assemble the hardware needed:

   - clear glass bowl, without any markings (remember the surface of the water needs to be covered with flowers if using them, so unless the flowers are big, get a small bowl). Cheap glass is usually the easiest to find and the best.

   - unbleached coffee filter paper

   - a small funnel is useful

   - water (not tap)

   - pre-sterilised bottle at least 30 mL.

2. Decide what the essence is to be made of and make sure:

   - there are enough flowers, leaves etc. can be obtained

   - permission has been given from the plant to use the flowers or other material (intuit/dowse/muscle test).

3. On a sunny day:

   - recheck that permission has been given

   - fill the bowl about half full of water

   - carefully pick enough flowers to cover the surface

- leave the bowl in full sunlight (remember that shadows move during the day), make sure it is safe from children, animals etc.

- check with a pendulum how long the essence needs to be left, or leave for about three hours.

4. When the time is up, return to the essence and dowse/intuit to see whether it is ready.

5. Bring the essence into a safe place and remove the flowers carefully from the bowl.

6. Filter the water into another clean container.

7. Fill the bottle at least 60–70 per cent with alcohol (ideally vodka or brandy 40 percent proof minimum).

8. Fill the remaining 30–40 per cent of the bottle with your flower essence water. This bottle becomes the mother essence. Label this bottle with the flower and date (and maybe the time). If this is kept this in a cool place away from electrical sources, it will keep for years.

9. If an option to charge the essence has been chosen, use a method to charge the mother essence before storing it.

CLEANSING MINERALS, CRYSTALS OR GEMS

New stones, providing they are not water soluble or too fragile, benefit from washing in warm, soapy water to remove dust and grime. But more importantly, all stones should be energetically cleansed before and after each use. Crystals will tend to carry vibrational patterns of all the people who have handled them on their way to personal ownership, so need thorough cleansing.

The lattice structures of crystals absorb and transform imbalances in their surroundings but they can quickly overload if not given the opportunity to be cleansed.

Ways to cleanse crystals

- **Running water and sunlight.** Hold stones under running water, visualising imbalances flowing away. Then place in sunlight to dry (not suitable for water-soluble crystals, fragile crystals or crystals that fade in sunlight).

- **Sound.** Sound vibrates matter. A singing bowl, bell, cymbal or tuning fork are very efficient energetic cleansers of crystals when held near to them.

- **Incense smoke.** Incense has always been used to cleanse and consecrate. Pass the stones several times through the smoke. Be aware of smoke alarms!

- **Salt.** A traditional remover of negativity. Avoid salt water as it corrodes crystals surfaces. Use dry sea salt to cover crystals overnight.

- **Breath.** Take a deep breath and exhale sharply over the crystals. Imagine imbalances being blown away. Repeat several times.

- **Crystal clusters.** Placing stones on larger crystals clusters, like clear quartz or amethyst, helps to restore natural levels of energy.

- **Essences and sprays.** Combinations of flower and gem essences can be used in an atomiser to cleanse crystals.

A 'clean' crystal feels different from an energetically 'tired' stone.

FLOWER ESSENCES CHALLENGE CURRENT UNDERSTANDING OF THE PLACEBO EFFECT

Michael E. Hyland PhD, CPsychol, Professor of Health Psychology, University of Plymouth

Many scientists assume that flower essences work as a kind of placebo effect. There are data supporting this view, as there have been a couple of blinded, randomised control trials that have failed to show a difference between placebo and flower essence. Although these data are limited, they lead to the conclusion that the mechanism underlying flower essence is that of a placebo. The principal mechanism underlying the placebo effect is that of expectancy. That is, someone expects to get better and so gets better. The reason why this expectancy then has a therapeutic effect is unknown. However, expectancy is the only plausible placebo mechanism that can explain the effect of flower essences (the other placebo mechanism, that of conditioning, does not apply in this context).[1]

Abstract

Objective

The aim of this study was to determine whether absorption and spirituality predict the placebo response independently of expectancy.

---

1   The full report of this research can be found at www.jpsychores.com/article/ S0022-3999(05)00214-X/abstract, accessed on 27 July 2014.

Method

This was an open study of self-treatment with self-selected Bach flower essences. Participants' expectancy of the effect of flower essences, attitudes to complementary medicine, holistic health beliefs, absorption and spirituality were measured prior to treatment. One month after the start of treatment, participants responded to an email enquiry about symptom change using a single seven-point change scale.

Results

A total of 116 participants (97 university undergraduates and 19 staff) completed all assessments. Spirituality and absorption together predicted additional variance compared with a cluster of expectancy measures comprising expectancy, attitude to complementary medicine, and holistic beliefs (increment in R^2 = .042, P = .032), and spirituality alone (but not absorption alone) predicted more additional variance than did the expectancy cluster (increment in R^2 = .043, P = .014).

Conclusion

Our data are inconsistent with conventional explanations for the placebo effect. The mechanism underlying the placebo response is not fully understood.

Acknowledgements: This research would not have been possible without the help of Sue Lilly, who co-ordinated and obtained materials for us, which were donated by Ainsworths, Healing Herbs, and Homoeopathic Supply Company free of charge. We thank Dr Andrew Tresidder for training in flower essence dispensing. The data were collected by three of my final year undergraduate students: Adam W.A. Geraghty, Oliver E.T. Joy, and Scott I. Turner.

APPENDIX 4

AUDIO ESSENCES

Brian Parsons

Ever since Dr Abrams created his first radionics machine at the dawn of the 20th century, the world of energy healing has been stubbornly growing, provoking a debate (in the minds of those who choose to listen) about what is actually required for healing and transformation to occur.

My contribution to this debate has been the development of Audio Essences.

My starting point was the assumption that an essence is created using three distinct elements – a vibration to be recorded, a medium upon which to record and transmit the vibration and an energy source used to imprint the vibration upon the medium.

So a traditional water-based essence is made using water as the recording medium, sunlight as the energy source and a crystal or flower as the vibration to be recorded. Although Audio Essences also uses three elements, two of these are quite different from the water-based approach.

The crystal or flower is the same, but the medium used to record the vibration is an MP3 file, and the energy source used to imprint the vibration on to the sound file is a Light-Life Ring, created by an American named Slim Spurling.

The resulting MP3 'transmission track' is then edited and merged into a music track, and the specific vibration can then be accessed whenever someone listens to that Audio Essence.

Now, I know that Audio Essences work for the majority of people, because they have been trialled on many different people, over the past couple of years, since their original creation. However, what isn't so easy is to explain how they work.

Because, if I were a traditional water-based essence producer, I could explain how they work through talking about the many wonderful and unique properties of water... But, unfortunately, water is not used as the medium of transmission in an Audio Essence, so that doesn't 'hold water'.

Well, perhaps I could explain about how sound can also influence our personal energies, but the actual transmission track, which is merged into the music, is completely silent. There are no sounds, tones or audible frequencies captured, so that doesn't work either.

After exhausting all the possible 'suspects', I have been forced to conclude that alongside the three elements of medium, vibration and energy source, there is also a fourth element involved in the essence creation process, and I have a feeling that this is also true for water-based essences (i.e. the ghost in the bottle).

Now, something which has always interested me is what is actually happening when something doesn't work, because if you pay attention when something doesn't work, you have the possibility of learning something new.

So it is very gratifying when someone reports that they have benefitted from listening to an Audio Essence, but the major leaps forward in their development have been through engaging with those people who said they weren't getting anything, and identifying why this was so.

Through working with such people, I have learned how an individual can block a vibration, and also how these energy blocks can be overcome, allowing the vibration to move deeper and deeper within their energy system.

But through doing this, I have concluded that real transformation only happens when a vibration touches something deep within us. And this 'something' is not located in our brain, or on the level of our 70 per cent puddle of water. I have come to feel it lies much, much deeper than that. Now, I am always wary of New Age practitioners who reach out into the world of quantum physics for a justification of their particular brand of 'magic'. However, through working with different essences, Audio Essences and the water-based kind, I have come to believe that this fourth element is consciousness itself, and that real transformation occurs when the essence vibration is able to touch this, our innermost consciousness.

APPENDIX 5

THE GATEWAY VISUALISATION

A gateway of some kind is perhaps the simplest image to use for indicating the movement from one perception to another, and, very often, nothing else is required. Because it is a quick transition, however (simply stepping over the threshold into another place), it does usually need quite a vivid portrayal to give enough 'boost' to the journeyer to move into the space beyond.

In practice it seems the type of doorway is unimportant: a simple curtain will do as well as an ironbound oak door. What is important is to hold the image as sharply as possible. It is a barrier and also a means to pass through into another world. In order to get to your desired destination, intent and a visual cue is needed.

Whatever you wish to explore – the nature of a tree or spirit, for example – you must take time to build a strong image superimposed upon the door of something that represents that thing, the goal of the journey.

To journey to the cherry tree spirit, a bunch of cherries could be imagined there in front of you, upon the door's surface, or a familiar cherry tree you know so well a clear image can be held. What is used is less important than the connection the visualiser makes with the image. If the thought of cherry always brings to mind a bowl of custard, then use that image. We are signalling to the unconscious, the deep mind, that this is our destination. The clarity and strength of the image will help the focus the experience.

Very often, because linear time is left behind, the visualiser finds themselves beyond the door before the conscious mind has constructed the opening and walking-through sequences. If this happens, simply go with it. Where personal conscious control is still in place, the next step after visualising the door and the sign of destination or purpose is to clearly intend your goal along the lines of, 'I wish to... (go to place or spirit)... and I ask permission to enter... (repeating the intended goal).' Clearly see the doorway opening in front of you and place yourself so that you are on the threshold.

Take a single step with as much awareness as possible, passing over the threshold and stand still. Allow time to register what it is that you are perceiving.

Go through all your senses in turn. What do you see? What do you feel? What do you hear? If you have not been immediately whisked away into scenes and landscapes, you may feel it appropriate to call for a guide to lead you to where you need to go.

Some people will enter fully into this Otherworld whilst others may just watch scenes unfolding from their vantage point at the doorway. What occurs is less important than recognising the significance of what occurs. When you are ready to return, will yourself back to the doorway, pass through it, turn around to visualise it as you did at first – closed firmly shut with no sign or image upon its surface.

Bring the attention back to the body and allow the imagery to fade away. Record impressions and experiences immediately. It is a good idea to write clearly the purpose of the journey before you start and then record experiences underneath.

Putting the actual words down on paper can help to clarify the events and prevents you from changing the parameters by altering the nuance of wording.

WHAT IS WELLNESS?

What is wellness? Maybe wellness is a state where the person considers they have no symptoms of dis-ease? Maybe wellness is a state where the person has symptoms of dis-ease but those symptoms are not considered to impact on the quality of life?

When a client brings symptoms to a session, what is the focus? Should the focus be the symptoms that are recognised? Should the focus be the underpinning issues of the person, as a whole?

If the focus is only on the symptoms and none of the underlying issues addressed, will the symptoms re-occur when the stress levels increase?

If the focus is only on the underlying issues, will the client get satisfaction from the session? Will the client understand the approach?

The diagram in Figure A6.1 shows a simplified idea of what can happen with a client.

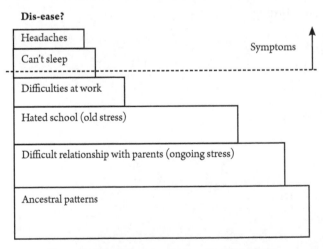

FIGURE A6.1 What can happen with a client

The boxes represent the underlying stresses. The line running through 'can't sleep' is the threshold between wellness and dis-ease. When the stress boxes exceed the threshold, symptoms are noticed. People have a tendency to have individually 'favourite' stress boxes at the top of the pile. These will show the recurring symptoms that are a nuisance and that wreck the quality of everyday living.

If the top of the pile of stress boxes drops below the threshold, noticeable symptoms abate.

The new client comes to a session suffering from headaches. It emerges in the session that they are also having difficulties sleeping. (These are the symptoms shown by the two top boxes.) Underlying these symptoms are several layers of stress – difficulties at work, a hatred of the times spent at school, difficulties with parents and some ancestral patterns, each with their own box.

The practitioner might choose to only focus on the symptoms so that the headaches and sleep difficulties will ease. In other words by taking essences these two boxes might then have been reduced enough in size to take the client's stress levels below the symptoms threshold. There would be much appreciation and praise from the client – problem sorted!

However, the next time the client has a bad day at work or a row with the parents (and those particular boxes of stress increase in size), it is likely the headaches would return, maybe even the sleep problems too. Great for maintaining a steady client flow, but maybe not really holistic care.

This particular diagram also explains what can happen if the client decides to go to a counsellor to deal with the family issues. The size of that stress box would then decrease dramatically and the headaches and sleeplessness go away, as their 'boxes' would consequently drop below the 'symptom' line.

Even more interesting, the diagram can also explain the situation where the client has already gone to a nutritional therapist about the headaches. The nutritional therapist dealt with that 'diet' box so well that the box is no longer there. However, the client feels the treatment did not work as the headaches are still present. If the headaches are then eased by essences the client thinks 'diet and supplements are rubbish, but those essences sure do work!' The nutritional therapist, when they get feedback from their client, might think – why didn't the nutrition changes work? The point being that it did but nutrition will not get the credit for it.

For argument's sake if the essence practitioner not only looked for essences to help with the headaches but also to deal with ancestral patterns, both the 'headaches' and the 'ancestral' stress boxes could be reduced in size. This would give rise to the second diagram.

Here the underlying stresses have been dealt with to such an extent that not only do the symptoms disappear but the client has gained some reserve to deal with future stresses.

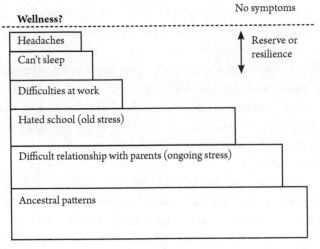

FIGURE A6.2 The underlying stresses have been dealt with

BIBLIOGRAPHY

Bach, E. (1931) *Heal Thyself.* Saffron Walden, UK: CW Daniel.

Bach, E. (1933) *The Twelve Healers.* Saffron Walden, UK CW Daniel.

Barnard, J. (2002) *Bach Flower Remedies, Form and Function.* Hereford, UK: Flower Remedy Programme.

Connelly, D.M. (1994) *Law of the Five Elements.* Laurel, MD: Traditional Acupuncture Institute.

Department for Business Innovation and Skills (2012) *Guidance: Product Safety for Manufacturers.* Available at https://www.gov.uk/product-safety-for-manufacturers, accessed on 13 October 2014.

Diamond, J. (1985) *Like Energy.* New York, NY: Dodd, Mead & Co.

Gerber, R. (2001) *Vibrational Medicine.* Rochester, VT: Bear & Co.

Gurudas (1983) *Flower Essences and Vibrational Healing.* Boulder, CO: Cassandra Press.

Gurudas (1985) *Gem Elixirs and Vibrational Healing Vol. I.* Boulder, CO: Cassandra Press.

Gurudas (1986) *Gem Elixirs and Vibrational Healing Vol. II.* Boulder, CO: Cassandra Press.

Hix, S. (1998) *Fourteen Classical Meridian Charts.* Grantham, UK: Rosewell Publications.

Hyland, M. (2005) *Spirituality predicts outcome independently of expectancy following flower essence self-treatment.* Plymouth, UK: School of Psychology, University of Plymouth.

Karim, I. (2010) *Back to a Future for Mankind: Biogeometry.* Self-published (CreateSpace).

Kröplin, B. (2005) *The World in a Drop.* Barcelona, Spain: CIMNE.

Lilly, S. (2002) *Modern Colour Therapy.* Johannesburg, South Africa: Caxton.

Lilly, S. and Lilly, S. (1999a) *Tree: Essence of Healing.* Taunton, UK: Capall Bann.

Lilly, S. and Lilly, S. (1999b) *Tree: Essence, Spirit, Teacher.* Taunton, UK: Capall Bann.

Lilly, S. and Lilly, S. (2004) *Tree Seer.* Taunton, UK: Capall Bann.

Lilly, S. and Lilly, S. (2001) *Colour Therapy.* Leicester, UK: Lorenz.

Lilly, S. and Lilly, S. (2001) *Chakra Healing*. Leicester, UK: Lorenz.

Lilly, S. and Lilly, S. (2006) *The Essential Crystal Handbook*. London, UK: Duncan Baird Publishers.

Pulos, L. (n.d.) *Positive and Negative Healing* available at http://drpulos.com, accessed 27 July 2014.

Schiff, M. (1995) *The Memory of Water.* London, UK: Thorsons.

Titchiner, R., Staines, P., Potter, R. and Monk, S. (1997) *New Vibrational Flower Essences.* Welling, UK: Waterlily Books.

Wheeler, F.J. (1952) *The Bach Remedies Repertory.* Saffron Walden, UK: CW Daniel.

Wiand, L. (2010) 'Bernard Grad, the legacy lives on.' *Subtle Energies and Energy Medicine* 21, 2.

USEFUL LINKS

Simon and Sue Lilly

Online Shop: www.greenmanshop.co.uk
(Essences, books, courses)
Courses: www.mcscourses.co.uk
(MCS Flower Essence Practitioner, ICGT Crystal Therapist training etc.)
Personal essence service: www.suelilly.co.uk

BFVEA

British Flower and Vibrational Essences Association – www.bfvea.com
Listing of essence practitioners, annual Gathering, 'Essence' journal.

Brian Parsons

www.audioessences.com

BAFEP

British Association of Flower Essence Producers: www.bafep.com
Listing of over 50 producers, multi-search Essence database.

COREP

The Confederation of Registered Essence Practitioners.

COREP is a collaborative venture between the two main essence professional bodies, The British Flower and Vibrational *Essences* Association (BFVEA) and The Bach Centre (www.bachcentre.com), and serves as the knowledge base for the practice of essence therapy in the UK: www.corep.net

FES

The Flower Essence Society recognises the importance of establishing a solid foundation of research for the development of flower essence therapy. In addition, the Flower Essence Society sponsors and assists controlled scientific studies on flower essence therapy: www.flowersociety.org